Canadian Health Care and the State

/93 ⫞

© McGill-Queen's University Press 1992
ISBN 0-7735-0934-8 (cloth)
ISBN 0-7735-0949-6 (paper)

Legal deposit third quarter 1992
Bibliothèque nationale du Québec

Printed in Canada on acid-free paper

This book has been published with the help of a
grant from the Hannah Institute for the History of
Medicine.

Canadian Cataloguing in Publication Data

Main entry under title:
  Canadian health care and the state

Includes bibliographical references.
ISBN 0-7735-0934-8 (bound). –
ISBN 0-7735-0949-6 (pbk.)
1. Medical care – Canada – History – 20th century.
2. Medical policy – Canada – History – 20th century.
3. Insurance, Health – Canada – History. I. Naylor,
C. David (Christopher David), 1954–
RA395.C3C265 1992   362.1′0971   C92-090364-9

This book was typeset by Typo Litho composition inc.
in 10/12 Palatino.

Canadian Health Care and the State

A Century of Evolution

EDITED BY C. DAVID NAYLOR

McGill-Queen's University Press
Montreal & Kingston • London • Buffalo

Contents

Special Acknowledgment

This collection of essays had its early origins in a seminar series on "Medicine and the Welfare State" organized in the spring of 1982 by Professor Pauline M.H. Mazumdar of the Institute for the History and Philosophy of Science and Technology at the University of Toronto. Dr Mazumdar had noted a paucity of secondary sources that dealt with the changing face of medicine and health services as the Canadian welfare state took shape. Her hope was that the seminar participants might contribute essays that could then be compiled into a useful academic source. Not all participants were able to transform their presentations into academic essays; hence the project had to be set aside. Dr Mazumdar asked the current editor to revive the collection in 1987, and lent the project additional impetus in 1987–88 by canvassing new contributors for essays and offering editorial commentary on some of the material at hand. Competing priorities and commitments precluded her continued participation in the editorial process, but the editor wishes to record his special thanks to Pauline Mazumdar for her role in this project.

Acknowledgments

In a collection of essays with a long gestation, numerous debts accumulate and I apologize in advance to those who should be acknowledged here but have somehow been overlooked. My first vote of thanks, of course, is to the contributors who have weathered various delays, multiple peer-review processes, and assorted editorial interventions. A specific thank-you must go to Susan Kent Davidson, who copy-edited the collection meticulously and insightfully on a short timeline. Philip Cercone, Peter Blaney, and Joan McGilvray at McGill-Queen's University Press shepherded the book through the review and production process in their usual professional and helpful fashion. Several of the anonymous referees offered constructive and detailed comments on the collection, and thereby emboldened this occasionally craven editor. I am also grateful for logistical help from Larry Stevenson of the Sunnybrook Clinical Epidemiology Unit at Sunnybrook Health Science Centre.

Dr Robert Macbeth, former director of the Hannah Institute for the History of Medicine, was supportive and patient when the final product did not meet prescribed deadlines.

Canadian Health Care and the State

Introduction

C. DAVID NAYLOR

Canadian health-care historiography is in the throes of a renaissance. The hallmarks are plain: new journals, organizations, and gatherings; more and better books and articles; increasing numbers of established historians and social scientists directing their attention to the field; and, as heralded by the notices of theses completed, a new generation of academics emerging who will focus on medical historiography from the outset of their careers.

Until the last several years, most of the work published was in three broad categories: biography or autobiography; "house histories" of professions, hospitals, faculties, and professional organizations; and sketches of important scientific developments.[1] These early publications have generally fallen within the paradigm of narrative historiography. While one should not underestimate the usefulness of a common-sense analysis of the flow of ideas and events, the narrative paradigm has limitations. It illustrates key themes but may lack the necessary analytical framework to interpret and illuminate events more fully.

Even in work published more recently the organizing principle has sometimes been either a Whiggish view of history as the unfolding of scientific and social progress or a simplus chronology. Better publications reflect a more sophisticated stream within this narrative tradition, drawing insights from sociological and political theory, philosophy of science, epidemiology, and health-services research. The best of these flesh out an analytical and thematic skeleton with relevant historiographic evidence, while others punctuate a chronology with analytical asides and thematic commentary. The overall impression remains that Canadian medical historiographers have been applying and honing the analytical tools developed elsewhere.

Three collections of essays have appeared in the last decade, providing the general reader with a sampling of work in this field. The first, edited by S.E.D. Shortt, was published in 1981 and drew primarily on articles published in the 1960s and 1970s (although one contribution had actually appeared in 1938 and another was new). *Medicine in Canadian Society* was in essence a chrestomathy, illustrating the range of the discipline and some of the more interesting contributions to it.[2] Shortt's introductory essay was a critical overview of previously published work, highlighting the potential for Canadian historians to explore the health-care field. The next major collection, *Health, Disease and Medicine*, edited by C.G. Roland, drew on papers presented at the First Hannah Conference on the History of Medicine (June 1982).[3] Like the Shortt volume, this collection was thematically eclectic, but it had the advantage of presenting work that had not previously been published. It illustrated the growing development of a professional and academic historiography of Canadian medicine. The latest collection, *Essays in the History of Canadian Medicine*, was edited by W. Mitchinson and Dickin McGinnis, both of whom contributed articles.[4] This 1988 volume was eclectic but contained seven original contributions of high calibre, exemplifying the trend to a more analytical and theoreticallly informed approach to our medical past.

The present collection of essays is offered as a further sampling of recent work in the social history of Canadian health care. In contrast to the previous three collections, there is a certain degree of thematic unity in that the essays were solicited to offer reflections on an issue of recurring interest – the modern origins, institutional manifestations, and effects of state involvement in the health-care field. Two essays on military medicine are included in light of the parastatal position of the armed forces. The authors, all present of former academics, are at different stages of their careers and come from a variety of backgrounds. Their training and academic accomplishments range across history, social science, and clinical disciplines. The topics and approaches are similarly varied. Some essays are snapshots of a given period; others are overviews covering several decades of development. Some cleave closely to the tradition of narrative historiography; others have a more analytical thrust, drawing on sociological theory or addressing policy issues.

As noted by Colin D. Howell in the opening essay, state mediation in the health-care services marketplace is often portrayed in terms of the agendas and tactics of competing private-interest groups. This paradigm has definite explanatory power, particularly for more recent decades, but – as Howell cogently argues – it fails to address the broader issues of class formation and the role of the professions in the rise of the modern welfare state. In Howell's essay the career and views of the Maritime medical doctor and social critic Alexander Peter Reid serve as a sounding-board for these themes.

The latter years of the nineteenth century saw unprecedented urbanization and industrialization. Faced with social upheaval as manifested by the disease-ridden working poor of Halifax and other urban centres, Maritime doctors were forced to consider "the various maladies of the body politic." Alexander Reid was a pillar of the Nova Scotia medical establishment and founding dean of the Dalhousie Medical Faculty. During the 1870s Reid began developing a vision of social reform that he was to expound repeatedly and persuasively for two decades. His book *Poverty Superseded: A New Political Economy for Canada* (1891) criticized unfettered capitalism and laid down the theoretical foundations for a benevolent government in which professionals would control the state apparatus. Inter-class conflict was to be reduced; competitive individualism would give way to expert management, and scientific principles would be applied to maximize the health and wealth of all citizens. This optimistic view of the state, allied with a strong belief in the social responsibility of professionals and experts, was eventually to gain widespread acceptance during the Progressive era in North American politics.

Howell's essay hints at more critical views of state mediation in the medical-services marketplace. One thinks here of P. Starr's multifaceted exploration of the professionalization process in American medicine, which dealt, among other things, with the conflict between the ideology of professionalism and traditions of communal and personal self-sufficiency in matters of health and disease.[5] While numerous essays have been written on professionalization in Canadian medicine, the only full-length study is by R. Hamowy.[6] His work is grounded in a libertarian critique of professionalism and therefore offers a detailed overview of the political and legislative developments that led to the closing of the Canadian medical-services marketplace. However, there remains a clear need for a full-length study of the rise of the Canadian medical profession that will marry historical and sociological analysis of the phenomenon of professionalization.[7] Indeed, while midwifery has received careful attention,[8] major analytical histories of health professions other than medicine have not appeared.

Reid's thought, with its overtones of social and eugenic engineering, was not atypical of the period. Angus McLaren's 1990 collection, provocatively entitled *Our Own Master Race*, provides ample documentation of this impulse as it evolved through and beyond the so-called Progressive period in Canada.[9] Howell's essay also implies that the welfare state was a way for the profession-technician stratum of society to augment its influence and abet social reform without more radical upheaval. There has been detailed exploration of medicine's historical position as handmaiden to the emergence of "compassionate capitalism" from a quasi-Marxist perspective elsewhere, yet little work of this nature has been done in Canada.[10] Unfortunately, in the social sciences and humanities it sometimes seems as if mixing and matching theoretical frameworks is considered a mark of bad taste or inadequate intellectual discipline. My own hope is that Canadian medical historians will avoid expending undue energy in arguing that one given theory is exclusively correct rather than accepting that sociological and historical phenomena are too complex to be captured under any single theoretical umbrella.[11]

Desmond Morton's contribution on "Military Medicine and State Medicine" reviews the experience of the Canadian Army Medical Corps in the First World War – the practice and politics of medicine in a difficult new environment. Close to half of Canada's active medical practitioners were in the corps, dealing with problems that bore scant resemblance to those of civilian medicine. The patients were relatively healthy young men, afflicted with sexually transmitted diseases or suffering from battle wounds, both physical and mental. Socio-economic change accompanied these clinical challenges as an occupational group composed of independent professionals was shaped into a disciplined state medical service with a clear hierarchy and salaried remuneration. How did this experience change the outlook of Canadian practitioners? And to what extent did the expanded role of the state in wartime health services carry over into the post-war period?

As documented by Morton, the changes wrought were important. The public-health challenges of the barracks and trenches provided a whole generation of Canadian doctors with an understanding of preventive medicine and what was then called "hygiene." This impetus spilled over into the post-war development of fields such as industrial and occupational medicine. The new sanatoria for soldiers helped to transform tuberculosis treatment from a charitable to a state concern, and the fear that returning soldiers would bring an epidemic of sexually transmitted disease sparked a nation-wide movement to compulsory treatment. However, the wartime flush of enthusiasm for radical reorganization of medical care quickly passed. The squabbles and patronage resulting from the marriage of military medicine and civilian politics created an understandable scepticism in the ranks. In Morton's view the returning soldiers had "experienced the collectivism of military life and a particularly oppressive form of socialized medicine" and were eager to stake their claim to civilian rewards rather than to change the society they had just defended.

In a narrative contribution drawn from his 1990 monograph *Battle Exhaustion*,[12] Terry Copp describes the development of neuropsychiatry in the Canadian army overseas during the Second World War. Parallels with the First World War are obvious: service in the armed forces brought doctors under the control of a parastatal authority, forcing upon them discipline and a complex bureaucratic system unlike any other organization they would encounter in peacetime. As had been the case in the Great War, there were questionable methods of examining volunteers and inadequate responses by many military authorities to the problem of neuropsychiatric disability stemming from battlefront trauma.

Copp's cast of characters includes many pioneers in Canadian neurology, neurosurgery, and psychiatry who were involved with the No. 1 Neurological and Neurosurgical Hospital at Basingstoke, England. Disagreements among the various specialists highlight the shaky scientific basis of psychiatry in the 1930s and 1940s. Much of the debate centred on an issue that was as much strategic as clinical: should the "psycho-neurotics" be excluded from active service and sent home, or was it worth expending scarce medical resources in an attempt to rehabilitate them? The Basingstoke hospital served as a training centre for many influential clinicians and academicians. The Canadian operation was also deemed highly successful by other Allied doctors, not least because the medical staff was able to impose its own priorities on the military bureaucracy.

Both contributions on military medicine are drawn from periods of international war. The same is true of the standard books offering histories of military medicine in Canada.[13] What remains little explored is the nature of military medicine in peacetime. Who have been the physicians, nurses, and other professionals functioning in the military environment? How did they differ from their colleagues in civilian practice, and why did they choose the military route? How has the military dealt with the potential attraction of private practice for its physicians? What prepayment arrangements have been put in place to ensure soldiers some free choice of physician and hospital? And what of the role of the military practitioners as agents of social control? Some of this latter function is captured in the essays by Morton and by Cassel in relation to sexually transmitted diseases, and Copp's essay implies that wartime psychiatry performed a similar function. Elsewhere, T. Brown's exploration of the treatment of shell-shock in the Great War not only analyzes differences in treatment by class and rank but also suggests that putting troops back into action was an adjunct to psychiatry's quest for respectability as a specialty. [14] Even in peacetime, one presumes, there are similar conflicts between the military practitioner's Hippocratic imperative as patient advocate and the role of health services in supporting the hierarchical structures and values of the military apparatus. In sum, much more needs to be known of how civilian and military medicine have differed through the decades.

Judith Young reviews the role of the state in a different light in her essay on the effects of socialized medicine and changing attitudes on class distinctions at the Hospital for Sick Children in Toronto from 1930 to 1970. Young's essay focuses primarily on the visiting policies of Canada's oldest pediatric hospital, finding that poor and working-class parents had limited access to their children, hospitalized on the "public wards," compared to those whose children were in private or semi-private beds. The psychological drawbacks of separating sick children from their parents were understood by the 1940s and 1950s, yet "Sick Kids" persisted in its restrictive policy. The spread of private insurance plans and eventual implementation of state-sponsored health insurance contributed to the blurring of distinctions between "public" and "private" patients, thereby abetting the overdue changes in visiting policies. This contribution illustrates how narrow historiographic keys can unlock wide doors, for it sheds light on broader issues such as class prejudices in health care, the formulation of hospital policy, and the impact of prepayment plans on patients and families.

Young's essay is also welcome because, of all the areas of Canadian medical historiography, the general hospital remains one of the least explored. [15] Thus far, we have had numerous histories of single institutions, which sometimes speak more to the self-importance of the hospital and its staff than to anything else. Disorganized summaries, often amounting to brief chronologies for each major institution, have also been published as part of older volumes that attempted to provided a global overview of health care (usually construed only as doctors, hospitals, and epidemics) on either the national or provincial fronts. One full-length volume appeared fifteen years ago, outlining some of the changes in the hospital sector between 1920 and 1970, but this was a labour of love by a pioneering physician-administrator rather than an academic overview informed by modern historiographic techniques.[16] Perhaps the only area that has had thorough analysis is the organization of prepayment for hospital services under private and public insurance plans.[17] Beyond that, one searches in vain for Canadian works that would parallel the many monographs that have illuminated our understanding of the role of the hospital in American and European societies.

We come next to a series of papers that bring a historical perspective to some facet of Canadian health services. The first of these, by Stephen J. Kunitz, offers an American's perspective on socialism and social insurance in the United States and Canada, with particular reference to the public health-insurance movement. Whereas Canada and the United States are often deemed similar in their adherence to classical liberal ideals, Canada has taken a radically different course in so far as state-sponsored prepayment of health services is concerned. Kunitz's essay offers an exploration of the various hypotheses advanced to explain the contrasts in ideology and social structures between the two nations.

Kunitz reviews the evolution of state health insurance in the United States, including the conclusions drawn by the factions of the famous Committee on the Costs of Medical Care in the 1930s. The opposition of the American Medical Association to health insurance at this time extended beyond state-sponsored prepayment to include any form of insurance, private or public, even though medical incomes were ravaged by the Great Depression. By the late thirties the American union movement had gathered momentum and was pressing actively for social-insurance measures. The unions, however, were only one voice in the liberal interest-group coalition that formed the voting block for the American Democratic party. Canada's third party, the Co-operative Commonwealth Federation, had a social-democratic ideology and strong commitment to public health insurance. The CCF-NDP in Saskatchewan was able to press forward with various state-sponsored prepayment measures, and their programs served as a catalyst for developments nationally. America eventually did implement a program of health insurance for the poor and aged but has since made little progress in public reorganization of the health-services marketplace. However, issues of equity and universal access, submerged during the Reagan years, seem to be on the American public agenda yet again as the 1990s begin.

Kunitz's arguments bring to mind Carolyn Tuohy's outstanding essay on "Conflict and Accommodation in the Canadian Health Care System."[18] It is of interest that, from opposite sides of the forty-ninth parallel, these two scholars have independently arrived at similar perspectives on the ideological and political forces at work in shaping North American health services.

Complementing Kunitz's essay is Eugene Vayda and Raisa Deber's overview of the contemporary Canadian health-care system. Health-administration experts with an interest in the historical evolution of Canadian health care, Vayda and Deber outline the political context and changes that have led to our present system, and offer an analysis of possible future developments. This is a substantially revised version of an article first published in *Social Science and Medicine* in 1984.[19] Both there and again in this essay, the authors warn that our publicly funded health-care programs are moving into an untenable financial position. Pressure for higher fees and incomes in the health-services sector, unchecked consumer demand, new drugs and technologies, and latterly a reduction in federal contributions have made it difficult for the provinces to afford their portion of the national health-insurance program. Thus, while Canada has successfully struck a balance between the American and British paradigms for health-service delivery, that balance that will be increasingly difficult to maintain.

The third overview essay is by Jay Cassel, author of *The Secret Plague*, a major monograph on venereal disease in Canada from the mid-nineteenth century to the outbreak of the Second World War.[20] In this contribution Cassel brings his readers up to date with a thorough review of government measures to control sexually transmitted diseases (STD) in the twentieth century. Contemporary concern with the acquired immunodeficiency syndrome (AIDS) gives Cassel's work an obvious relevance.

It rapidly emerges from Cassel's study that the "magic-bullet" philosophy has pervaded government policy for decades. From 1917 to 1983, by far the largest part of public expenditure on STDs went towards medical measures; the figure seldom dropped below 85 per cent of the total allocations by federal and provincial governments. As Cassel argues, these spending priorities effectively limited public-education programs, contact tracing, and individual-patient counselling services. There has also, until recently, been an abysmally low level of funding for STD research.

Cassel's historical perspective brings to light many recurring themes in the Canadian campaigns against STDs. In both world wars "loose women" were blamed for the transmission of venereal disease. The prevailing epidemiological view was that a few women infected many men and that men were to be excused for promiscuous sexual activities because of their supposedly stronger sex drive. Obviously the tendency to seek scapegoats for STDs continues today. The pricing and distribution of drugs for STDs has caused repeated difficulties, manifested most recently in the controversy over the costs of supplying azidothymidine (AZT) for the treatment of AIDS. Educational programs, too, remain fragmented and flawed. Through the years Canadians have been unrealistically enjoined to abstain from sexual activity, or given information about STDs so lacking in basic details as to have little impact on sexual practices. Public piety has seldom been reflected in private sexuality, yet policies to deal with STDs have often been shaped by the moral prejudices of the day rather than a realistic appraisal of human behaviour. In short, Cassel's work has a number of lessons for the public, policy-makers, and professionals. It will also be useful for scholars because of its extensive bibliographical references.

The last of the overview essays is again one with many contemporary messages and is of methodological interest because of its interdisciplinary framework. Robin Badgley and Samuel Wolfe raise discomfiting questions about the goals and achievements of Canada's state-sponsored health-insurance system. As documented by the authors, the continuing links between low income, limited education, and ill health have been repeatedly demonstrated in this nation for a half-century. During the Depression social reformer Leonard Marsh led a study that warned against reliance on a medical model to deal with health problems rooted in socio-economic conditions. The 1951 Canadian Sickness Survey confirmed the presence of substantial inequity in health care: low-income citizens had poorer health and consumed significantly fewer medical services. None the less, it is evident from the essay by Badgley and Wolfe that policy-makers were oriented to treating the diseases of poverty rather than attacking poverty per se.

The medicare debate in Canada was driven by the optimistic belief that elimination of economic barriers would automatically guarantee equality of access to health care, and that equality of access in turn would lead to equality of health status. Badgley and Wolfe review a series of studies over the last twenty years that have attempted to address the validity of those assumptions. In all, about two dozen reports have dealt with the issue of social class and health-service utilization. The bulk of these studies restrict themselves to the analysis of a single service, and many do not distinguish between the types and quality of services. Analysts have focused simply on visits and expenditures without considering the overall health status of the poor or comparing expenditures across social classes for patients matched by diagnoses and severity scales. Statistical and conceptual pitfalls abound: for example, factors such as family size may be ignored in relating service consumption to household income, and the co-variation of income, education, needs, and health status renders interpretation of results difficult. In fact, the most methodologically rigorous reports have suggested that there remains a positive or direct relationship between income level and average health-insurance benefits received.

The Honourable Marc Lalonde's *New Perspective on the Health of Canadians* (1974) gave federal ministerial recognition to the limits of the medical model for dealing with illness, and in 1987 the Honourable Jake Epp's ministry followed suit in calling for a health-promotion approach that might reduce class inequities in health status.[21] However, these words have never been translated into economic or political action. Indeed, the fiscal framework of medicare continues to stint on federal support for provinces most in need of assistance. The current move to reduce federal contributions to health care will only exaggerate these regional inequities. Badgley and Wolfe do not tell us how to resolve these problems, but they wed historical, epidemiological, and political analysis in demonstrating how and where Canada's cherished medicare program may have failed precisely those underprivileged persons it was designed to assist.

Whatever the future holds in terms of the pattern of institutionalization of health services in Canada, health-care historiography is now emerging as an exciting field of research and analysis that can offer useful insights. The social history of medicine cannot, of course, offer up ready-made solutions to present-day problems. Historiography instead illuminates trends, occasionally highlights pitfalls that should be avoided in future, and invariably offers the consolation of learning that, while actors and backdrops change, certain plots are played out repeatedly as the decades roll by. Indeed, the enduring lesson of history may be that social change is inevitable and institutional progress possible, but human nature is wonderfully intransigent.

NOTES

1 Useful bibliographies are to be found in two other collections of essays. See W. Mitchinson and J.D. McGinnis, eds., *Essays in the History*

of Canadian Medicine (Toronto: McClelland and Stewart 1998), 198–218; and S.E.D. Shortt, ed., *Medicine in Canadian Society: Historical Perspectives* (Montreal: McGill-Queen's University Press 1981), 495–506. A more exhaustive bibliography is C.G. Roland, *Secondary Sources in the History of Canadian Medicine* (Waterloo: Wilfrid Laurier University Press 1985).

2 See n 1.

3 C.G. Roland, ed., *Health, Disease and Medicine: Essays in Canadian History* (Toronto: Hannah Institute for the History of Medicine/Clarke Irwin 1984).

4 See n 1.

5 P. Starr, *The Social Transformation of American Medicine* (New York: Basic Books 1982).

6 R. Hamowy, *Canadian Medicine: A Study in Restricted Entry* (Vancouver: Fraser Institute 1984).

7 There are any number of American and European sources that offer either examples of the genre or theoretical insights applicable to writing such a study. A few of those commonly cited are Starr, *Social Transformation*; M.S. Larson, *The Rise of Professionalism* (Berkeley: University of California Press 1979); T.J. Johnson, *Professions and Power* (London: Macmillan 1972); J.L. Berlant, *Profession and Monopoly: A Study of Medicine in the United States and Britain* (Berkeley: University of California Press 1979); and N. Parry and J. Parry, *The Rise of the Medical Professional: A Study of Collective Social Mobility* (London: Croom Helm 1976). Indeed, we have yet to replicate the detail and insights found in some American sources that are not twenty years old – e.g. W.G. Rothstein, *American Physicians in the Nineteenth Century: From Sects to Science* (Baltimore: Johns Hopkins University Press 1972). None the less, simply by drawing together published articles and other secondary-source materials, and stitching them together with a sociological framework, one could take a major step towards filling some of the scholarly void that persists.

8 See, for example, S. Buckley, "Ladies or Midwives? Efforts To Reduce Infant and Maternal Mortality," in L. Kealey, ed., *A Not Unreasonable Claim: Women and Reform in Canada, 1880–1920* (Toronto: Women's Press 1979), 131–49; various papers in *Ontario History* 75, no. 1 (Mar. 1983), especially C.L. Biggs, "The Case of the Missing Midwives: A History of Midwifery in Ontario from 1795–1900," 21–35; V. Strong-Boag and K. McPherson, "The Confinement of Women: Childbirth and Hospitalization in Vancouver, 1919–1939," *BC Studies* 69/70 (Spring/Summer 1986): 142–74; and generally, K. Arnup, A. Levesque, and R. Roach Pierson, eds., *Delivering Motherhood: Maternal Ideologies and Practices in the 19th and 20th Centuries* (London: Routledge

1990), particularly the essay by H. Laforce on midwifery in Quebec (36–50).

9 A. McLaren, *Our Own Master Race: Eugenics in Canada, 1885–1945* (Toronto: McClelland and Stewart 1990).

10 See E.R. Brown, *Rockfeller Medicine Men: Medicine and Capitalism in America* (Berkeley: University of California Press 1980). A recent overview of Marxist theories applied specifically to the medical profession can be found in V. Navarro, "Professional Dominance or Proletarianization? Neither," *Milbank Quarterly* 66, supp. 2 (1988): 57–75. Canadian contributions include D. Swartz, "The Politics of Reform: Conflict and Accomodation in Canadian Health Policy," in L. Panitch, ed., *The Canadian State: Political Economy and Political Power* (Toronto: University of Toronto Press 1977), 311–43; and A. Moscovitch and J. Albert, eds., *The Benevolent State: The Growth of Welfare in Canada* (Toronto: Garamond Press 1987).

11 W.L. Wallace, "Overview of Contemporary Sociological Theory," in W.L. Wallace, ed., *Sociological Theory: An Introduction* (Chicago: Aldine Publishing 1969), 1–59.

12 T. Copp and B. McAndrew, *Battle Exhaustion: Soldiers and Psychiatrists in the Canadian Army, 1939–1945* (Montreal: McGill-Queen's University Press 1990).

13 W.R. Feasby, ed., *Official History of the Canadian Medical Services, 1939–1945*, vols. 1 & 2 (Ottawa: Queen's Printer 1953, 1956). J.G. Adami, *The War Story of the CAMC, 1914–1915: The First Contingent* (Toronto: Musson Book Company 1919). H.A. Bruce, *Politics and the CAMC* (Toronto: William Briggs 1919).

14 T. Brown, "Shell Shock in the Canadian Expeditionary Force, 1914–1918: Canadian Psychiatry in the Great War," in Roland, *Health, Disease and Medicine*, 308–32.

15 See, for example, S.E.D. Shortt, "The Canadian Hospital in the Nineteenth Century: An Historiographic Lament," *Journal of Canadian Studies* no. 4 (Winter 1983–84): 3–14. Many of the same complaints could be raised about the evolution of general hospitals in the first half of this century.

16 G.H. Agnew, *Canadian Hospitals, 1920–1970: A Dramatic Half-Century* (Toronto: University of Toronto Press 1974).

17 Several sources discuss hospital insurance. Among the monographs are M.G. Taylor, *Health Insurance and Canadian Public Policy: The Seven Decisions That Created the Canadian Health Insurance System* (Montreal: McGill-Queen's University Press 1978); C. Howard Shillington, *The Road to Medicare in Canada* (Toronto: Del Graphics 1972); and C.D. Naylor, *Private Practice, Public Payment: Canadian Medicine and the Politics of Health Insurance, 1911–1966* (Montreal: McGill-Queen's University Press 1986).

18 C. Tuohy, "Conflict and Accommodation in the Canadian Health Care System," in R.G. Evans and G.L. Stoddart, eds., *Medicare at Maturity: Achievements, Lessons and Challenges* (Calgary: University of Calgary Press 1986), 393–434.
19 E. Vayda and R. Deber, "The Canadian Health Care System: An Overview," *Social Science and Medicine* 18 (1984): 191–7.
20 J. Cassel, *The Secret Plague: Venereal Disease in Canada, 1838–1939* (Toronto: University of Toronto Press 1987).
21 J. Epp, *Achieving Health for All: A Framework for Health Promotion* (Ottawa: Health and Welfare Canada 1987); printed as a supplement to the *Canadian Medical Association Journal*, 1 Mar. 1987.

Medical Science and Social Criticism: Alexander Peter Reid and the Ideological Origins of the Welfare State in Canada

COLIN D. HOWELL

The development of the modern welfare state, and more particularly the introduction of state-supported health insurance, is often seen in relation to the divergent intentions of competing interest groups. Such has been true of most treatments of the coming of medicare to Canada, where the competing and often shifting attitudes of organized labour, health reformers, politicians, medical organizations of various types, and civil-service bureaucrats are dissected in order to explain the timing of medicare's introduction.[1] What is often missed in this approach is the relationship between state involvement in health matters, the emergence and rising authority of the scientific professions, and the involvement of those professions in movements for social and economic reform. In this sense the roots of state medicine can be found in the nineteenth century, particularly in the liberal reform impulse commonly referred to as progressivism.

An amalgam of various elements, progressivism involved a faith in a scientifically rationalized and efficient capitalist system that would be able to overcome the abuses and social dislocations of too-rapid industrialization.[2] Professionals of various kinds took a leading role in the turn-of-the-century reform movement, asserting their expertise in the management of social problems and calling for a reorganization of society in accordance with new notions of scientific orthodoxy.[3] Faith in scientific management and professional expertise permeated the reform of politics, municipal government, criminal justice, labour relations, and industrial production,[4] and extended to the field of medicine and public health as well.[5] Furthermore, as Howard Segal has argued in his *Technological Utopianism in American Culture*, the progressive belief in science and social engineering stimulated a vision of a utopian society that would promote efficiency and social co-operation, place technical expertise above partisan political authority, and eschew wasteful individualism.[6]

This paper investigates the relationship between professionalization, progressive reform, and state intervention in the late nineteenth-century Maritimes by examining the career of medical doctor and progressive social critic Alexander Peter Reid. An asylum and hospital superintendent, public-health advocate, and a leading figure in the professionalization of medicine in the Maritimes, Reid pursued a career that sheds light on the relationship between medical professionalization, the veneration of scientific knowledge, and the promotion of sanitary, social, and moral reform. It should be noted at the outset that no claims are made here that Reid was typical of the rank and file of the medical profession; he was instead a member of that profession's own elite, many of whom were, like him, proponents of progressive social reform. At the same time Reid's commitment to a new and somewhat utopian social order – which could be achieved, he believed, through social planning and expert management – lent credibility to the idea of greater state involvement in matters involving the nation's mental, moral, and physical well-being.

Modern urban and industrial capitalism came to the Maritimes in the last third of the nineteenth century, fuelled by railroad and mineral development and the protectionist policies of the Canadian state.[7] As was true elsewhere, rapid industrialization and urbanization focused public attention on a wide range of social issues, from the living conditions of the poor to crime, prostitution, alcoholism, disease, child labour, women's rights, mental hygiene, and public sanitation. Doctors soon found themselves offering advice upon the sanitary condition of factories, schools, and tenements, the need for pure water, milk, and unadulterated food, the value of playgrounds and other recreational facilities, and the need for city sewers and refuse collection. Hitching a faith in science to a progressive concern for social improvement, many doctors began to envisage a hygienic utopia administered by a cadre of professional experts and appropriately trained agents of the state. What were needed, argued the progressive politician Dr J.B. Black of Windsor, Nova Scotia, were federal and provincial departments of health fully equipped with inspectors, sanitary engineers, bacteriologists, and chemists, assisted by city, town, and county boards of health with their own appropriately salaried officers. "When governments, national, provincial, and municipal, properly undertake the prevention of preventable disease," Black wrote, "then shall preventable diseases disappear from the civilized world."[8]

As the late nineteenth-century medical profession became more interested in questions of public health and sanitation, doctors gradually came to realize that their own social utility extended beyond the treatment of disease into a consideration of the various maladies of the body politic. Concerned that the rapid advance of civilization was contributing to the increase of nervous disorders, sexual debility, and moral degeneracy, doctors in the Maritimes – like their counterparts elsewhere – served up a coherent interpretation of social deviance and what had to be done to eradicate it.[9] In the process the hygienic utopia of the late nineteenth-century medical profession took on the character of a moral utopia as well, extending beyond the public-health movement to a broader interest in social and moral regeneration. Applying what they considered appropriate scientific remedies to social dislocation, doctors like Reid hoped to rid society of the "degenerative" influences of crime, insanity, gender conflict, and class antagonism and to replace competitive individualism with a blend of social co-operation and technical expertise.[10] Implicit in this progressive reform vision was a critique of traditional institutions such as the church, the family, and the old-line political parties, which were seen to have failed to address the abuses of the modern industrial order. The involvement of medical doctors in the progressive movement thus contributed to the medicalization of concerns that hitherto had been the province of the family, the church, the institutions of criminal justice, and the patronage-based party system, and represents an early first step in the direction of the modern therapeutic and capitalist welfare state.[11]

Alexander Peter Reid was one of the most articulate and prolific exponents of this vision of progressive reform and social regeneration in the late Victorian Maritimes. A committed scientist whose career spanned the half-century between Confederation and the First World War, Reid was convinced that the application of scientific and therapeutic principles to the social body would liberate mankind from the irrationality of modern urban and industrial society and fulfil hopes for a prosperous and disease-free future. Jettisoning the doctrines of survival of the fittest, competitive individualism, and retributive justice in favour of the corporate and therapeutic ideology of the welfare state, Reid remained a life-long proponent of the practical utility and applicability of science to daily life. Like other technological utopians, of course, he overestimated the extent to which modern science and technology could address the problems that science and technology had helped to create. Instead he shared the fanciful vision of Benjamin Ward Richardson, who in a memorable address to the Health Section of the British Social Science Association in 1875 fashioned the mythical "Hygiea," a disease-free urban utopia supervised by a hierarchy of medical officers, registrars, sanitary inspectors, chemists, and scavenging personnel.[12]

Reid's belief in the practical value of science and the importance of professional expertise in solving social problems stemmed from an early education that rejected the notion of "knowledge for its own sake." Born in London, Ontario, on 22 October 1836, Reid attended a private school in London until the age of twelve, when his father, a Scottish artisan who had emigrated to Upper Canada during the 1820s, took him out of school, complaining that he was not learning enough of practical benefit. Upon leaving school Alexander worked alongside his father as a cooper's assistant and pursued his education on his own. Picking out the subjects to be proficient in – Latin, algebra, geometry, and Greek – the young Alexander spent his unoccupied time in the morning and evening preparing for a useful career. In 1845 he enrolled in the Faculty of Medicine at McGill University, graduating four years later with the faculty's *materia medica* prize for his thesis on strychnia.

After graduation Reid spent a year of further study in Britain, returning to Canada in 1859 to practise medicine in Exeter and Clanboye near London, Ontario. Apparently, however, a rural practice in a frontier environment provided an insufficient challenge to Reid's scientific inquisitiveness and restless curiosity, and in the following year he closed his practice and began a journey across the continent and back. Travelling first to the Red River Settlement in the North-Western Territory, he dabbled in natural science, collecting information on skunks and the migration patterns of birds that formed the basis of a number of papers presented subsequently to the Nova Scotia Institute of Science. In 1861 he left the prairies for the Pacific coast, following it south to California. Although the American Civil War had already begun, Reid continued his travels, arriving in New York City sometime in 1862, where he undertook studies that led to another degree in medicine. In 1864 he journeyed to Halifax, and for the next fifty years he was a leading actor in the professionalization of medicine and psychiatry and a tireless advocate of closer ties between the state and the medical profession in public-health and social-reform matters.[13]

Reid arrived in Halifax in the midst of a movement to upgrade the professional and scientific status of the region's doctors. During the 1850s and 1860s the medical elite of Halifax was engaged in a program of professional self-improvement and reform that included the development of a provincial medical society (1854) and – with state assistance – the establishment of the Nova Scotia Hospital for the Insane (1859), the opening of the City and Provincial Hospital (1867), and the refinement of existing medical legislation. Within a few years of arriving in the city Reid had become a prominent figure in the Halifax medical fraternity. He was a founding member of the Scientific Branch of the Halifax Medical Society in 1867, gained notoriety as the first proponent of the germ theory in Nova Scotia, and was founder and president of the Clinical Society of Halifax, established in 1869. His other pursuits included efforts to legalize dissection (resulting in the Anatomy Act of 1868), assistance in drafting the legislation of 1872 that gave the medical profession the right to self-regulation, and participation in the founding of the Dalhousie Medical Faculty in 1868 (subsequently the Halifax Medical College). Reid was the first dean of the faculty and later president of the Halifax Medical College, and held successively the chairs of physiology, practice of medicine, hygiene, and medical jurisprudence.[14]

Reid's continuing interest in the application of scientific knowledge to the management of society led him in 1878 to apply for and accept the position of superintendent at the Nova Scotia Hospital, usually referred to as the Mount Hope Asylum. Already exhibiting many of the assumptions of the late nineteenth-century progressive, including faith in progressive education and an antipathy to sectarian animosities, Reid referred in his letter of application to his long-term interest in the "progress of education," his opposition to unfortunate and unscientific religious sectarianism, and his attraction to the asylum as a laboratory for social reform. Asylum administration was a particularly significant vocation, he observed, because no other area within medicine offered a wider field for human observation or greater promise for developing scientific principles upon which a new social order could be established. Indeed, Reid's work at the hospital over the next decade and a half provided him with the opportunity to develop therapeutic principles that could be applied both to the treatment of the insane in Nova Scotia and more generally to the reshaping of Canadian industrial capitalism.[15]

In appointing Reid as superintendent, the province revealed its own interest in having the asylum run in a more efficient, businesslike, and scientific manner. Reid's predecessor at the hospital, Dr James R. DeWolfe, had been removed from his position after a commission of inquiry in 1878 raised questions about the treatment of patients under his care. DeWolfe also came under fire for providing liberally for his family, who lived with him on the hospital grounds.[16] Ironically, DeWolfe had at one time been a reformer in his own right. A graduate of Edinburgh Medical School, an institution widely noted for its humanitarian attitudes and its reliance upon moral treatment as an alternative to more Draconian forms of incarceration, DeWolfe regularly impressed upon his staff the virtues of non-restraint of the insane and the therapeutic value of work, religious instruction, and recreation. Other than this articulation of general principles, however, DeWolfe tended to let the institution run itself. His subordinates were not encouraged to bring specific concerns about the operation of the hospital before him, and his medical assistant, Dr Fraser, was once reported not to have conferred with DeWolfe for over four years. In the end the report of the commission occasioned a complete dismissal of all senior staff at the asylum, and led in turn to Reid's appointment as superintendent.[17]

Reid's approach to the treatment of the insane was very much in line with that of other North American asylum superintendents, who regarded hereditary predisposition and physical imperfections in the brain as the major causes of insanity. Concerned that moral treatment had no scientific basis and that asylum superintendents without a scientific therapeutic orientation were essentially indistinguishable from prison wardens, many late-nineteenth-century alienists sought a plausible scientific rationale for treatment that would both legitimize the profession and help to cure the insane. In search of a scientific explanation for insanity, therefore, Reid adhered to the prevalent somatic theory, which suggested that derangement originated in lesions of the brain or spinal cord. Like many of his contemporaries he attributed mental illness to physical disorders "of the higher ganglia of the nervous system ... most frequently in their minute structure," the capillary vessels.[18] Just as the germ theory suggested the specificity of disease and hence of therapeutics, Reid believed that medical science eventually would be able to predict a particular lesion with a given case of insanity. Once that was done, the mental hospital would be in a position to establish effective therapy and liberate society from the burden of insanity. The institutionalization of the insane and the advancement of science would have served a social purpose: the cured would return to the workaday world normal and well adjusted.[19]

Unfortunately, the relationship between physical disorders and mental derangement could not be demonstrated scientifically. No matter how much asylum superintendents like Reid sought a somatic rationale for therapy, asylum care remained custodial. Somatic theory did little more than legitimize existing managerial techniques.[20]

The therapeutic limitations of somaticism, moreover, help to explain Reid's continuing reliance on moral treatment during the 1880s, despite his growing discomfort with its seemingly unscientific basis. In his first *Annual Report* for the year 1878 Reid had outlined the kind of therapy generally provided at Mount Hope. Treatment included manual labour (including work in the garden or on the hospital farm, ditch digging, plastering, painting, and cleaning) and exercise and recreation (including walking, music and dancing). Although religious instruction was usually a major component of moral treatment, Reid made no mention of it. Instead, he emphasized the need to acquire funds to improve the library, decorate the walls, and furnish improvements.[21] There is little indication that Reid's approach to treatment at Mount Hope changed over the next decade.

Reid did not rely totally on moral treatment of the insane, however. Like many of his contemporaries elsewhere in North America he also advocated mild forms of restraint, which, he believed, would protect the insane from self-injury and ensured a more placid asylum community. Where James DeWolfe had relied upon solitary confinement and sedation to control potentially violent patients, Reid employed restraining devices such as the "muff," a canvas or leather muff secured to the hands, armless jackets and dresses, crib beds, and strong canvas bedcovers, calling restraint a necessary activity that "the higher faculties must exercise over the baser ones inherent in our common humanity." Mild restraint also served as an alternative to physical force, which, "if used with sufficient energy to keep a patient overpowered ... [the patient] suffers in many ways, of which broken ribs are not infrequent forms." It also rendered unnecessary both the use of sedatives, "which deaden or weaken rather than strengthen or benefit the debilitated nervous system," and solitary confinement, in which the abnormal imagination might conjure up fearful phantasms and frightful delusions.[22] In Reid's mind the role of the superintendent was to protect the insane from their own self-destructive tendencies with a minimum amount of physical coercion.

The notion that the weakest members of society had to be protected from themselves and prevented from undermining social cohesion was a recurring theme not only in Reid's therapeutic approach to insanity but in his larger social vision. To Reid insanity and mental weakness implied biological degeneracy, which, if left untreated and unmanaged, would retard social progress and the advance of civilization. Furthermore, in order to treat the insane and to ensure social improvement, it was essential to recognize the importance of heredity in human behavior. In Reid's view the prime factor in cases of insanity was hereditary predisposition,[23] which posed particular problems for a province experiencing the initial incursions of modern industrial capitalism, as Nova Scotia was during the 1880s. Among other things, the demographic shift from countryside to town and city strained existing family units, reduced the respect for traditional forms of work, threatened the dignity of labour, altered gender relations, and set class against class. As Reid and like-minded progressives saw it, the great classes, held in organic harmony for centuries, were now being pulled asunder by the coming of industrial capitalism. What is more, the massive exodus from the Maritimes of those who could not be absorbed into the new industrial economy contributed to further social instability. Reid believed that this outmigration, which began in the 1870s and took on significant proportions in the years before the First World War, siphoned off those with the strongest nervous systems and thus exerted a degenerative influence on the province as a whole. Mental weakness, he argued, had been introduced into Nova Scotia from the "old countries" by the parent stock. Furthermore, because those with weak nervous systems lacked the drive "that impels the 'pushing class' ... [to] go to foreign or distant parts to better their condition," they would stay in the province and continue to pass on their mental weakness to their offspring. Nova Scotia's insane population was thus bound to increase. Asylums would be forced to extend accommodation for the insane in an increasing ratio "until society solves the problem of how to prevent its natural increase."[24]

Reid's hereditarian ideas led him gradually to lose faith in the asylum's curative potential. As these institutions became filled with chronic patients, occupying spaces designed to accommodate those more amenable to treatment, effective treatment suffered. Overcrowding of this sort, of course, was a difficulty common to all asylums. In London, Ontario, Dr Richard Maurice Bucke, an acquaintance of Reid's, treated recent and chronic cases in separate buildings, as did a number of institutions in Britain and the United States.[25] Reid advocated the introduction of this widely touted "cottage system" to Nova Scotia and called in turn for an elaborate system of county asylums that would receive chronic patients and allow the provincial asylum to concentrate on those cases where the chances of successful treatment were higher. Unfortunately for Reid, the Nova Scotia government was then facing a severe fiscal crisis and could not act on his suggestions. County asylums were not developed in the province until the late 1880s.[26]

Reid's disillusionment with the therapeutic limitations of the asylum led him ultimately to propose a broader plan for dealing with the country's "unfit," "degenerate," "weak," and "impecunious" population. Although this plan included many objectionable suggestions, it none the less embodied a progressive faith in scientific management and social engineering. Reid argued for an alliance between the state and the scientific professions to regulate excessive competition in the marketplace and to provide the "respectable" poor with appropriate protection from exploitation and disease. A reformed social order, Reid believed, should include a system of marriage control or eugenics to stem social degeneracy, a greater involvement of the state in public-health matters, and a revamping of the existing capitalist system to eradicate destructive class conflict. Reid's blueprint for this new social system appeared in various medical periodicals, in a number of papers read to the Nova Scotia Institute of Natural Science, and in the publications arising out of his later career in public-health administration.

Reid's late-nineteenth-century efforts to extend medical authority beyond concerns of health and disease and into non-medical matters such as marriage control or economic regulation helped to rationalize what Robert Nye has called "the intrusive medicalization of the twentieth century welfare state."[27] As Nye has pointed out, medical advice in the late nineteenth century was growing in public esteem: progressive politicians, administrators, and jurists – themselves imbibing a faith in scientific expertise – increasingly turned to doctors to prescribe remedies for social ills. In explaining and offering remedies for alcoholism, prostitution, juvenile delinquency, and venereal disease, moreover, doctors like Reid often turned to contemporary degeneration theory and the idea of hereditary transmission for their inspiration. Finding examples of social and moral degeneration wherever he looked, Reid suggested that sanitary practice, expert management of the economy, and a program of scientific breeding or eugenics would stem the decline.

One of the more comprehensive statements of Reid's progressive utopianism can be found in "Stirpiculture or the Ascent of Man," a paper read before the Nova Scotia Institute of Natural Science in January 1890 and published the following year in pamphlet form for wider public distribution. Addressing the many influences that could alter what he called the "culture of the race," Reid pointed out that horticulturists and stock-breeders routinely applied Darwin's evolutionary principles to the improvement of the stock, and suggested a series of "laws" that should be followed to ensure the "ascent of man." These included the prevention of hereditary transmission of defective characteristics; the sanctity of the marriage bond and its home associations; a correct appreciation of the dignity of labour;

moral training with fixed or positive religious ideas; a general and practical education; and definite instruction in sanitary laws. The first of these – the prevention of the hereditary transmission of congenital defects – was directed at what Reid called the "irresponsibles," which included the insane, the idiotic, and the criminal; the remainder were for the great bulk of humanity, those "moulded by ... association and learning."[28]

Reid's hygienic utopia involved isolating and eventually eradicating "deviance" through selective breeding and sterilization. Reliance on marriage control and eugenics, he believed, would reduce the incidence of crime, and allow for a more efficient distribution of the state's resources. In addition, it would protect children from being born with the sins of their parents inflicted upon them.[29]

In his support for marriage control and eugenics, Reid was taking a position that had widespread support among medical men in the Maritimes and elsewhere. For example, when Reid left the Nova Scotia Hospital in 1894 to assume the position of superintendent of the Victoria General Hospital in Halifax, a successor as asylum superintendent, William Hattie, quickly revealed himself to be a staunch advocate of "scientific" marriage. In addition to arguing for legal restrictions upon "the marriage of the unfit," Hattie cautioned parents to take a rational rather than a sentimental approach to their children's marriages. Arguing that debilitating conditions such as tuberculosis or arthritis in parents tended to result in a lack of vigour in the nervous organization of their children, Hattie called for "the sacrifice of self as opposed to the sacrifice of offspring." In most cases, Hattie believed, moral suasion would suffice to prevent "promiscuous" or unsafe marriage. In the case of the feeble-minded, however, Hattie called for the legal prevention of their right to marry.[30] Dr A.B. Atherton of Fredericton was even more outspoken than Hattie. In his presidential address to the Maritime Medical Association in August 1907 Atherton expressed a widespread turn-of-the-century concern about the declining purity of the race and called for legislation to prevent the marriage of "those who are defective in physical and mental or perhaps even moral qualities." Society, Atherton argued, has a right and a responsibility to prevent diseased or defective individuals from transmitting defective characteristics "to a rising generation." In Atherton's opinion the insane, the feeble-minded, the diseased, and the chronic criminal "should be required to submit to sterilization."[31]

Marriage control and eugenics had a particular attraction to public-health advocates and asylum superintendents in the Maritimes, most of whom called for preventive measures both to protect against disease and degeneracy and to ensure physical and mental hygiene. Dr G.E. Coulthard, secretary to the New Brunswick Board of Health, for example, deplored the lack of attention given to the fight against tuberculosis and called for the prohibition of consumptives from travelling on buses, coaches, and railways. At the same time, he was convinced that TB sufferers passed on a damaged constitution to their offspring, and called for restrictions on their right to marry. If law-makers could prohibit drinking, he argued, surely they "could say authoritatively that these persons should not marry."[32] Other public-health officials and asylum superintendents in the Maritimes, such as George L. Sinclair, William Bayard, James T. Steeves, James A. Steeves, George Hetherington, Edward S. Blanchard, J.V. Anglin, and V.L. Goodwin, held similar views. Anglin stressed the need for the state and the churches to refuse marriage licences or to perform marriages "except in cases where there is reasonable prospect of healthy issue proceeding from such a marriage." James T. Steeves noted the need to prevent "neurotic subjects from ... extending the volume of degeneracy down the path of human existence."[33] Similarly, Charlottetown's Dr Edward Blanchard, superintendent of the Prince Edward Island Hospital for the Insane, warned that insanity would increase as the struggle for living became more competitive and that the costs of sustaining the insane in institutions would eventually become prohibitive. Blanchard's solution was the complete asexualization of all who showed signs of mental and moral weakness.[34]

When pressed, advocates of the eugenicist solution defended their position as an expression of modern scientific principles, a necessary prerequisite to the new hygienic utopia. In supporting their case, moreover, they could draw upon the work of criminal anthropologists such as Cesare Lombroso, Enrico Ferri, Havelock Ellis, and Henry Maudsley, all of whom regarded crime as a symptom of degeneracy both in the individual and society. The most influential of these quasi-scientific treatises was Lombroso's *Criminal Man* (1876), which defined crime as a function of the partly pathological and partly atavistic personality. Lombroso described the criminal as an atavistic being who revealed in his or her anti-social behaviour the ferocious instincts of primitive man and the inferior animals. Lombroso's theory also undertook to explain the apparent "stigmata of degeneration," the enormous jaws, large ears, drooping eyelids, and asymmetrical facial features that signified a criminal personality.[35] At the same time Lombroso suggested the possibility of scientific intervention to halt social decline and to encourage social regeneration. Indeed, despite its reactionary characteristics, Lombroso's new "science" of criminal anthropology proposed to reform an antiquated, unscientific, and retributive criminal-justice system and replace it with a therapeutic and scientifically grounded legal system in which the expertise of the medical profession was essential.[36] Dr O.J. McCulley of Saint John, who shared Reid's progressive views and was an outspoken advocate of therapeutic justice, drew heavily upon Lombroso's writings. The criminal, wrote McCulley, "is morally infirm and we should treat him in the same spirit as we treat the physically infirm ... This must be done in no spirit of vindictiveness, with no mawkish sentimentality, but with scientific methods." These methods would be directed at transforming the criminal from an anti-social into a social being, and failing that, preventing the propagation of the criminal's kind, either through sterilization or capital punishment.[37]

Like many progressives who feared social degeneracy, Reid also remained convinced of the possibility of social regeneration. In particular he believed that the state and the educational system could encourage moral improvement by inculcating Christian principles, instructing in the duties of citizenship, protecting society from disease through regular instruction in sanitary laws, and developing a state-supported system of public-health administration. Predictably, Reid took a leading role in the development of Nova Scotia's public-health apparatus, assuming the position of secretary to the Provincial Board of Health in 1893. As the most active proponent of a progressive public-health system in the province he continually encouraged his colleagues to enter the political arena in order to secure "a thorough, systematic, well-trained, and well-paid sanitary department"[38] and demanded greater involvement at all levels of government, from the province to the county to the municipality. What was needed, he argued, was for doctors to emulate the legal profession, where judges not only sat in high courts but in "every corner." Largely because of Reid's campaign the provincial government abolished the Provincial Board of Health in 1903, replacing it with a Health Department under the provincial secretary and with a salaried executive officer known as the provincial health officer. Reid was the first to serve as health officer for the province, and continued in that position for another decade.[39]

Like many other progressive reformers in Canada and the United States, Reid's interest in the sanitary movement was coloured by a deeply-held nativist bias. Just as he had attributed the source of much mental weakness to people from the "old countries," Reid was convinced that immigration infected Canada with disease and class antagonism. In this he shared the sentiments of many of his colleagues, who believed that immigrants were usually from the "lower orders" and not only carried with them inherited or epidemic diseases but a "degraded moral nature derived from inherited tendency and criminal surroundings."[40] Canada, he believed, not only needed protection against insanity but against the degenerative impact of unrestricted immigration. In a paper in the *Maritime Medical News* for September 1899 entitled "Sanitary Progress," Reid drew upon a biblical analogy in order to demonstrate how prophylactic principles could result in the "uplifting of society." The mission of Moses, the law-giver, Reid argued, was to elevate his followers to a higher level, to turn an "ignorant, diseased, immoral, irreligious and effeminate" race of slaves whose highest ambitions were "the fleshpots of Egypt" into a liberated people. To achieve this objective a plan in "harmony with ... present knowledge" was applied. The Israelites were quarantined in the desert; the diseased were placed outside the camp and were prohibited communication with the healthy. Moses, Reid wrote, "took forty years to accomplish a journey easily made in forty hours, and this was the secret of his success." Because every individual who left Egypt, even Moses himself, died before the entry into the promised land, the new race was composed of individuals sprung from the best of the old stock brought up under the best sanitary surroundings, trained and educated, and made to conform to very strict sanitary regulations.[41] The point of this allegory is clear: Reid considered scientific expertise, immigration restriction, and an effective public-health apparatus essential to the process of social regeneration.

The final component of Reid's progressive reform vision involved the reconstruction of the existing capitalist system in accordance with the principles of scientific management, state regulation, efficient, production, and co-operative enterprise. Reid was particularly critical of an excessively competitive marketplace, which created a great gulf between wealth and poverty and led to destructive class conflict. At the same time he found business organization to be unscientific, irrational, and biased towards the powerful. In Nova Scotia, for example, the province's underdeveloped business class not only lacked technical and theoretical knowledge but, in competing with more industrialized areas, was rendered ineffective by its insufficient access to capital. Reid thus forecast limited industrial growth for the Maritime provinces in the future and argued for the exploitation of the natural advantages that the region had in its primary-resource sector. In a speech to the Dairymen's Association of Nova Scotia in 1890, for example, he outlined the problems confronting an inefficient regional dairy industry as it faced competition from large oleomargarine producers elsewhere in the country, and suggested the development of production and marketing co-operatives. "Experience has dissipated a fond delusion I had in the efficiency of joint stock companies," Reid wrote. "The capital is apt to be limited and as well uselessly dissipated by want of skill in the directorate board, or the promoters – technical ability is too apt to be measured by the number of friends the applicant may have on the board of directors." Instead, Reid favoured the co-operative ownership of the dairy industry by the producers themselves. These co-operatives could be established through the introduction of a toll system, in which a farmer would give a percentage of this raw material to the state in return for the capital required to produce and market dairy products.[42]

Some years earlier Reid had applied a similar analysis to the fishing industry, emphasizing the importance of state support and scientific practise in developing the resource. Fishermen who followed the practical man's "rule of thumb" in catching, curing, and selling fish, Reid argued, failed to appreciate the very important economic potential of increased scientific knowledge of the life-cycle, feeding habits, and food-chain of marine species. To improve the understanding of market conditions and to stimulate scientific research, Reid called for an academy of science – either state-operated or privately endowed – which would increase scientific understanding and "eliminate the theory of chance and the so-called bad years from the list of probabilities." In addition he advocated more emphasis on natural science in the school curriculum, called for greater state assistance in promoting an equivalent to agricultural co-operatives for the fishing industry, and proposed a marine aquarium that, in educating youth about the animals that contribute to the region's prosperity, would establish a foundation of "provincial greatness."[43]

In general Reid saw a future in which a benevolent state and a cadre of professional experts would put science before profit, thus replacing competitive individualism with expert management. The result would be economic prosperity, social justice, and class peace. This was the theme of Reid's *Poverty Superseded: A New Political Economy for Canada* (1891), which, in calling for a reorganization of the capitalist marketplace, laid down a rationale for the modern Canadian welfare state. Drawing heavily from both Henry George's analysis of the antagonistic character of progress in *Progress and Poverty* and the scientific utopianism of Edward Bellamy's *Looking Backward*, Reid began his study of existing political economy with a critique of competitive individualism and the emerging credit system. The inevitable result of the free market, he suggested, was inequality, for even if the economic race were adjusted to the point of equality, some would soon come to dominate it. Most individuals were skilled producers when operating under the guidance of skilled administrators, he believed, but few had the mental ability to command and direct economic affairs. As a small number of effective managers succeeded, therefore, their success encouraged others to enter into competition, which in turn led to diminishing profits and the failure of many businesses.

The difficulties faced by the weak in the competitive marketplace, Reid argued, led naturally to the emergence of the credit system, which he saw as a major social and economic evil. To Reid credit led to indulgence in unnecessary luxuries and encouraged the less judicious to live beyond their means. In the long run this would increase the difficulty of the debtor as it enhanced the power of the creditor. Taken together, competitive individualism and the credit system meant wealth for the few and poverty for the many. *Poverty Superseded* tried to address this dichotomy by having the state assume the care of the weak. Reid wrote:

Since the Government, local or general, must assume the care of the impecunious or incapable, it should have the right to direct to some extent the way the earnings of the community are disposed of, and this leads to the principle underlying Communism, a principle not so much questioned as the methods designed to carry it out. This is very well worked out by Bellamy in his *Looking Backward*, and also to a certain extent by Henry George in his *Progress and Poverty*. General Booth deals with this problem but his plan is rather adapted to relieve present want, immorality and crime than a method which would eliminate them.

In addition to abolishing laws providing for the collection of debts – which he believed would destroy the credit system – Reid suggested that the state be given the right to collect a percentage of the income of every wage-earner, male or female, which then would be placed to his or her credit at interest, dispensed by the state if the person needed relief. But if a person was required to set aside a percentage of his earnings, he asked, did it not follow that he or she should be assured a continuous means of earning? In Reid's view the state should be held responsible for ensuring full employment, and this could be achieved through the introduction of public works programs funded in part by the revenues collected from wage-earners. In this way, he argued, "the whole country ... would become a mutual benefit society."[44]

While arguing for a society run on co-operative principles rather than upon the doctrine of competitive individualism, Reid was none the less careful to point out that state regulation should not threaten the principle of private ownership of the means of production. In Reid's view the state should operate merely as a medium of regulation, transferring wealth to those who needed assistance. It was not desirable, Reid argued, that it interfere with or attempt to control the trade or business of the country in any way. In the case of industrial stagnation, however, the state could act as a reservoir into which surplus products would flow and from which they would then flow out again when a demand arose. At the same time government should be given the power to curtail production when the supply of particular commodities far exceeded demand, and be empowered to direct labour into some other channel. In this way the state would "relieve the misery which *strikes, lockouts,* or *clogged markets* impose on the wage earner."[45]

Reid's desire to have the state actively engaged in protecting the economic interests of the weak also led him to call for a government-sponsored system of general life insurance. This was by no means an original notion: Charles Tupper, for example, had once supported the idea but chose not to act upon it owing to the opposition of private insurance companies. Reid argued, however, that the good of society was of greater importance than the selfish interests of private capital. "The management of a country," he wrote, "cannot be run solely in the interest of these financial corporations." At present, Reid pointed out, it was only the well-off who patronized these companies, and they should be encouraged to continue to do so. It was the poorer classes who needed state protection. A government scheme, therefore, should insure applicants only to a necessary minimum level, thereby allowing for the continuing profitability of private companies.[46]

In calling for the remodelling of Canadian capitalism along progressive lines, Reid was convinced that he was transcending the class interests of capital, replacing competitive individualism with a more scientific, responsible, and benevolent social order. "So far society has depended upon the ability of the individual to manage the increasing mass of labour and as might have been expected the individual works chiefly for his personal gain," wrote Reid, "and wielding those powerful engines – capital and combination – the ideal state of society ... has been obliterated." The concentration of economic power in the hands of a few, moreover, carried with it the heavy price of enduring class conflict and interrupted production. Strikes paralysed society, and the capitalists reacted with violence to suppress workers. This kind of disorder, Reid concluded, would continue until "society as represented by Government, undertakes – I would say is forced to undertake – the regulation of industry."[47] It would be more than a decade, however, before the kind of progressive view of labour-management relations that Reid subscribed to would gain political currency in Canada. Even then the commitment to a tripartite resolution of labour disputes – one that involved the participation of the state, the business class, and labour and was enshrined in legislation like the Industrial Disputes and Investigations Act of 1907 – served the interests of capitalists more than it did those of working people.[48]

Although many of Reid's ideas – particularly his eugenicist notions – were never acted upon, his call for the reform of Canadian society along progressive lines reveals a growing belief in the need for a scientific solution to the problems besetting late nineteenth-century capitalist society.[49] In calling for the rehabilitation of the capitalist system, for an increased state involvement in public-health matters, and an increasing respect for the social value of professional expertise, Reid shared many of the assumptions of those turn-of-the-century progressive reformers who were discarding Spenserian notions of "survival of the fittest" in favour of the doctrine of social responsibility and moral regeneration. Reid's veneration of science, his faith in the wisdom of the medical profession, and his commitment to the medicalization of social problems that had long been the responsibility of other institutions, moreover, helped to shape his vision of a future hygienic utopia, free of poverty, crime, disease, and class antagonism.

Reid's progressive vision, which included a commitment to what Christopher Lasch has called the modern "therapeutic state,"[50] grew out of his work in medicine, the asylum, and the field of public health. His faith in medical science and its practical application led him to advocate an enhanced role for the professional expert in the articulation of social policy. His experience as an asylum superintendent was also important here, reinforcing his concerns about biological and social degeneracy and confirming his belief that the diseased society, like the diseased mind and body, needed the therapeutic intervention of the scientific practitioner. To Reid the eradication of mental disorder through selective breeding and eugenics was a scientific and even humanitarian policy, and like efficient public-health initiatives promised a hygienic and prosperous future. Reid's work and writings, like those of many reformers in the Maritimes and elsewhere, moreover, helped to shape the emerging progressive reform impulse and contributed to the emergence of that new managerial class of benevolent experts that attached itself to the developing welfare state. Unfortunately, Reid's faith in science "practically applied" led not to utopia but instead to the new form of expert management – often hostile to traditions of self-help and more radical forms of social criticism – that has accompanied the coming of welfare-state capitalism in the twentieth century.

NOTES

1 See, for example, C. David Naylor, *Private Practice, Public Payment: Canadian Medicine and the Politics of Health Insurance, 1911–1966* (Montreal and Kingston: McGill-Queen's University Press 1986); and Malcolm G. Taylor, *Health Insurance and Canadian Public Policy: The Seven Decisions That Created the Canadian Health Insurance System* (Montreal: McGill-Queen's University Press 1978).

2 Samuel P. Hays, *The Response to Industrialization: 1885–1914* (Chicago: University of Chicago Press 1957); Robert Wiebe, *Businessmen and Reform* (Cambridge: Harvard University Press 1962); Samuel Haber, *Efficiency and Uplift: Scientific Management in the Progressive Era* (Chicago: University of Chicago Press 1964); James Weinstein, *The Corporate Ideal in the Liberal State* (Boston: Beacon Press 1968). For Canada, see Robert Craig Brown and Ramsay Cook, *Canada 1896-1921* (Toronto: McClelland and Stewart 1974).

3 Burton J. Bledstein, *The Culture of Professionalism: The Middle Class and the Development of Higher Education in America* (New York: W.W. Norton 1976); Thomas Haskell, *The Emergence of Professional Social Science* (Urbana: University of Illinois Press 1977).

4 Samuel P. Hays, "The Politics of Reform in Municipal Government in the Progressive Era," *Pacific Northwest Quarterly* 55 (1964): 157–69; Stanley Schultz and Clay McShane, "To Engineer the Metropolis: Sewers, Sanitation, and City Planning in Late Nineteenth Century America," *Journal of American History* 65 (1978): 389–411; Reginald Whitaker, "The Liberal Corporatist Ideas of Mackenzie King," *Labour/Le Travailleur* 2 (1977): 137–69; Alfred Chandler, *The Visible Hand: The Managerial Revolution in American Business* (Cambridge: Harvard University Press 1977); H.V. Nelles, *The Politics of Development* (Toronto: Macmillan 1974).

5 George Rosen, "The Efficiency Criterion in Medical Care, 1900–1920," *Bulletin of the History of Medicine* 50 (1976): 28–44; Barbara Gutmann Rosenkrantz, *Public Health and the State: Changing Views in Massachusetts, 1842–1936* (Cambridge, Mass.: Harvard University Press 1972): Heather MacDougall, "The Genesis of Public Health Reform in Toronto, 1869–1890," *Urban History Review* 10, no. 3 (1982); and "Public Health and the 'Sanitary Idea' in Toronto, 1866–1890," in Wendy

Mitchinson and Janice Dickin McGinniss, eds., *Essays in the History of Canadian Medicine* (Toronto: McClelland and Stewart 1986), 62–87; Colin Howell, "Reform and the Monopolistic Impulse: The Professionalization of Medicine in the Maritimes," *Acadiensis* 11, no. 1 (Autumn 1981): 3–22.

6 Howard Segal, *Technological Utopianism in American Culture* (Chicago: University of Chicago Press 1985).

7 T.W. Acheson, "The National Policy and the Industrialization of the Maritimes," *Acadiensis* 1, no. 2 (Spring 1978): 3–28.

8 J.B. Black, MD, MP, "Race Suicide with Suggestions of Some Remedies," *Maritime Medical News* 19, no. 7 (July 1907): 248–9.

9 Robert A. Nye, *Crime, Madness, and Politics in Modern France: The Medical Concept of National Decline* (Princeton, NJ: Princeton University Press 1984). On the idea of degeneracy see Ruth Friedlander, "Benedict-Augustin Morel and the Development of the Theory of Degenerescence," PhD, University of California 1983; Richard Walker, "What Became of the Degenerate? A Brief History of a Concept," *Journal of the History of Medicine and Allied Sciences* 11, no. 4 (1956): 422–9.

10 There is no comprehensive treatment of the idea of degeneracy in Canada. Samuel E.D. Shortt, *Victorian Lunacy: Richard Bucke and the Practice of Late Nineteenth Century Psychiatry* (Cambridge: Cambridge University Press 1986), 99–103, provides a brief summary of the concept.

11 On the origins of the welfare state in Canada, see Allen Moscovitch and Jim Albert, eds., *The Benevolent State: The Growth of Welfare in Canada* (Toronto: Garland 1987).

12 J.H. Cassidy, "Hygiea: A Mid-Victorian Dream of a City of Health," *Journal of the History of Medicine and Allied Sciences* 17, no. 2 (April 1962): 217–18.

13 *Public Archives of Nova Scotia* (PANS) Verticle File, "Alexander Reid"; Henry Morgan, *Canadian Men and Women of the Time* (Toronto 1898), 850.

14 Colin D. Howell, "Elite Doctors and the Development of Scientific Medicine: The Halifax Medical Establishment and 19th Century Professionalism," in Charles G. Roland, ed., *Health, Disease, and Medicine: Essays in Canadian History* (Toronto 1984), 105–22.

15 Alexander Reid to Hon. P.C. Hill, Provincial Secretary, 29 Dec. 1877, PANS, Nova Scotia Hospital Records, RG 25A, vol. 16.

16 *Acadian Recorder*, 6 Apr., 15 May 1878.

17 Ibid., 11 Apr. 1878.

18 22nd Annual Report, Medical Superintendent, Nova Scotia Hospital, *Journals and Proceedings of the House of Assembly of the Province of Nova Scotia (JHA)* 1880, app. 3, p 5.

19 Ibid., 6–10.
20 L.S. Jacyna, "Somatic Theories of Mind and the Interests of Medicine in Britain, 1850–1879," *Medical History* 26, no. 3 (1982): 233–58.
21 21st Annual Report, Medical Superintendent, Nova Scotia Hospital, *JHA* 1879, app. 3, pp 4–6.
22 22nd Annual Report, Medical Superintendent, Nova Scotia Hospital, ibid. 1880, app. 3, pp 7–10.
23 25th Annual Report, Medical Superintendent, Nova Scotia Hospital, ibid. 1883, p 7.
24 25th Annual Report, Medical Superintendent, Nova Scotia Hospital, *JHA* 1883, p 7; Alan A. Brookes, "Out-Migration from the Maritime Provinces, 1860–1900: Some Preliminary Considerations," *Acadiensis* 5, no. 2 (Spring 1976): 26–55.
25 Cheryl Krasnick, "'In Charge of the Loons': A Portrait of the London, Ontario, Asylum for the Insane in the Nineteenth Century," *Ontario History* 74, no. 3 (1982): 143.
26 The fiscal crisis is dealt with in Colin D. Howell, "W.S. Fielding and the Repeal Elections of 1886 and 1887 in Nova Scotia," *Acadiensis* 8, no. 2 (Spring 1979): 28–46.
27 Nye, *Crime, Madness, and Politics.*
28 Alexander P. Reid, *Stirpiculture and the Ascent of Man* (Halifax: T.C. Allen 1890), 4.
29 Ibid., 6. The history of the eugenics movement is touched upon in a number of sources. See in particular Mark Haller, *Eugenics: Hereditarian Attitudes in American Thought* (New Brunswick, NJ: Rutgers University Press 1963); Donald Pickens, *Eugenics and the Progressives* (Nashville: Vanderbilt University Press 1968); Kenneth Ludmerer, *Genetics and American Society: A Historical Appraisal* (Baltimore: Johns Hopkins University Press 1972); Angus McLaren and Arlene Tigar McLaren, *The Bedroom and the State* (Toronto: McClelland and Stewart 1986); Charles Rosenberg, "The Bitter Fruit: Heredity, Disease, and Social Thought in 19th Century America," *Perspectives in American History* (Cambridge: Harvard University Press 1974), vol. 8, 189–235.
30 W.H. Hattie, "The Prevention of Insanity," *Maritime Medical News* 16, no. 2 (Feb. 1904): 41–8.
31 A.B. Atherton, "Presidential Address to the Maritime Medical Association," *Maritime Medical News* 19, no. 8 (July 1907): 247–54. Atherton even added cured tuberculosis patients to the list of those who should be prevented from siring children. "Even if cured," he asked, "why should they be allowed to bring children into the world who will inherit a ... pronounced tendency to the same disease?"
32 8th Annual Report of the Provincial Board of Health, New Brunswick, *Journals of the House of Assembly* 1895.

33 Report of the Medical Superintendent of the Provincial Hospital, ibid.
    1914.
34 Ibid. 1893.
35 Gina Lombroso Ferrero, ed., with an introduction by Cesare Lom-
    broso, *Criminal Man According to the Classification of Cesare Lombroso*
    (New York and London 1911). See also Henry Maudsley, *The Physiol-
    ogy and Pathology of Mind* (London: MacMillan and Co. 1867).
36 See, e.g., Enrico Ferri, *Criminal Sociology* (New York 1897).
37 O.J. McCulley, "The Doctor and the Criminal," Presidential Address
    to the Saint John Medical Society, *Maritime Medical News* 17 (Feb.
    1905): 41–53. McCulley's address, which received the unqualified en-
    dorsement of the Saint John Medical Society, included a long disquisi-
    tion on the physical indications of degeneracy and the hereditary
    predisposition to crime.
38 A.P. Reid, "The Relations of the Profession to Society," *Maritime Medi-
    cal News* 1, no. 5 (July 1889): 102–3.
39 "The Nova Scotia Public Health Association," *Maritime Medical News*
    19, no. 4 (Apr. 1907): 128; "The Public Health Act of Nova Scotia,"
    ibid. 18, no. 6 (July 1906): 216–20.
40 Dr Edward Farrell, "President's Address before the Annual Meeting of
    the Maritime Medical Association," *Maritime Medical News* 7, no. 8
    (1895): 162–3.
41 Alexander Reid, "Sanitary Progress," *Maritime Medical News* 2, no. 9
    (Sept. 1899): 301–8.
42 A.P. Reid, "The Dairy of the Future – or – Theory and Practise Com-
    bined," paper read before the Dairyman's Association, Halifax,
    18 May 1899 (Halifax: T.C. Allen 1890).
43 A.P. Reid, "Natural History of the Fisheries," *Proceedings and Transac-
    tions of the Nova Scotia Institute of Science, Halifax, Nova Scotia* 4, no. 2
    (1875–76): 131–6.
44 A.P. Reid, *Poverty Superseded: A New Political Economy for Canada* (Hali-
    fax: T.C. Allen 1891), 7.
45 Ibid., 10.
46 Ibid., 11.
47 Ibid., 15.
48 For a discussion of the impact of the IDIA on labour-management re-
    lations, see Ian Mackay, "Strikes in the Maritimes, 1901–1914," *Aca-
    diensis* 13, no. 1 (Autumn 1983): 40–3.
49 For a discussion of the growth of a scientific progressivism and its re-
    lationship to an earlier ethical and Christian progressivism, see David
    B. Danborn, *'The World of Hope': Progressivism and the Struggle for Ethi-
    cal Public Life* (Philadelphia: Temple University Press 1987); and
    Ramsay Cook, *The Regenerators: Social Criticism in Late Victorian Canada*
    (Toronto: University of Toronto Press 1985).

50 Christopher Lasch, *The Culture of Narcissism: Life in an Age of Diminishing Expectations* (New York: W.W. Norton 1978).

Military Medicine and State Medicine: Historical Notes on the Canadian Army Medical Corps in the First World War 1914–1919

DESMOND MORTON

1. MEDICAL CRISIS

In the wake of the First World War, insisted Dr J.L. Todd, McGill's professor of parasitology, "it will be unbelievably easy to achieve social ideals which before the war seemed impracticable and impossible of achievement."[1] A wartime major in the Canadian Army Medical Corps (CAMC), Todd was convinced that experience with military medicine would make a post-war system of state health insurance inevitable. Many of his fellow physicians in Canada and the United States agreed. Surely too many people had experienced a fully organized health system to go back to the old ways of individualism and neglect.

From August 1914, when the first volunteers hurried to enlist, to the "Last Hundred Days" of 1918, Canadian medicine was fully committed to a national war effort. A pre-war army medical corps of 23 permanent-force officers reached an establishment, by the end of the war, of 1,525 medical officers, 1,901 nursing sisters, and 15,624 other ranks. By the armistice in 1918, the CAMC managed 36,209 hospital beds overseas and more than 12,000 in Canada. Hundreds of Canadian doctors volunteered for the British Army or served with the French, Belgians, Serbians, and Russians. Fully 3,000 doctors, close to half Canada's active medical practitioners and most of the leaders of the professions, served in the war. An individualistic profession, clothed in the myth of equal competence, created from its ranks a salaried, disciplined state medical service, with status based on seniority and military performance.[2]

Nothing less could have met the wartime crisis. A nation creating its first mass citizen army would not have tolerated the suffering that Florence Nightingale found at Scutari or Canadians had seen for themselves in the fever hospitals of Bloemfontein in 1900. At the same time, the war Canada entered so blithely in 1914 created battlefield casualties at an unprecedented rate. Within a year of the outbreak France alone had to cope with a million war wounded. In the Canadian Expeditionary Force (CEF) 39,488 soldiers were killed in action and another 12,048 died of wounds; the medical miracle was that 154,361 survived their wounds and four out of five returned to active service.[3]

For the first time in a major war, death by enemy action took a heavier toll than death from disease. As recently as the South African War 64 Canadian soldiers had been killed in action while 71 died of sickness, 58 of them from typhoid fever. In the CEF 6,767 of 59,544 fatal casualties were due to disease, only 45 of them to typhoid.[4] Medical science, mobilized by the army, conquered some of the traditional slayers of armies. Army experience in turn suggested how a host of other problems, from disability to venereal disease, might be tackled by a civilized society. Todd's optimism about post-war medical reorganization was accordingly neither unfounded nor unique.

Of course the army was not everyone's model. Doctors in uniform chafed at regulations, resented less competent military superiors, and returned to civil practice with their individualism reinforced.[5] Soldiers were humiliated by the arrogance of medical officers more mindful of their status than their bedside manner. Military medicine emphasized the gulf between the physician and the "non-paying" patient and reinforced it with King's Regulations. If state medicine continued such military habits as early-morning sick parade, baring one's genitals for a "short-arm inspection," or swallowing the notorious Number 9 pill, many veterans had been successfully inoculated against it.[6]

2. ARMY MEDICAL CORPS

The CAMC owed its origins to Frederick Borden, Laurier's minister of Militia and a former militia surgeon from Nova Scotia. The improvised hospitals that sufficed for the North-West Campaign of 1885 or the couple of doctors a militia regiment added to its strength would not be adequate for the self-contained Canadian army Borden was bent on creating. In 1900 Borden authorized the first specific militia medical units. He also established that nurses, commissioned as lieutenants, would be part of the organization – forty-one years before the British Army followed suit.[7] Borden's reforms delighted the medical profession. A militia commission had long been a benefit to a struggling local practitioner, guaranteeing both respectability and a special contingent of patients. An army medical corps flattered the self-importance of the profession. In turn, doctors made their own contribution to Canada's pre-war drive for preparedness, from Dr Eugene Fiset, Borden's choice as deputy minister, to Colonel J.T. Fotheringham, the pillar of the Canadian Defence League.

When war came in 1914, the CAMC may well have been better prepared than other elements of the militia. It was needed at once to inspect recruits, vaccinate them, and (at least initially on an optional basis) inoculate them against typhoid.[8] Confident, like other volunteers, that the war would be brief as well as triumphant, doctors and nurses volunteered by the hundreds. Thanks to a British request for four additional hospitals and a casualty clearing unit, demand fortunately came close to matching supply. In England the CAMC survived its first crisis when an epidemic of spinal meningitis struck down hundreds of soldiers, most of them fatally. Recriminations between the Canadians and their British hosts faded to oblivion when the epidemic died away and most of the troops left for France as the First Canadian Division.[9] Some of the hospitals had preceded them.

It was apparent by then that the war would not be brief or glorious. The Canadians entered battle when the most desperate material shortages, including a lack of hospital cots and medical supplies, had been overcome, but they soon encountered the horrors of modern combat. At Ypres, in April 1915, the Canadians lost 6,714 of their 20,000 men. Medical services were overwhelmed by the horrible wounds inflicted by shellfire and the equally appalling effects of chlorine gas. In Captain F.A.C. Scrimger, from McGill University, the CAMC could boast its first Victoria Cross winner. In Colonel John McCrae, a gunner-turned-medical officer from Guelph, it had the war's first major poet.[10]

The heroic tradition was valuable, but experience and efficiency took longer to acquire. Like other permanent-force officers who shaped the expanding CAMC, Major-General Guy Carleton Jones owed his post more to Liberal connections than to medical standing, but he rose to the crisis. The Royal Army Medical Corps provided him with training and military medical doctrine. In turn, Jones and a few others could train Canadian doctors and orderlies in Britain methods.[11]

Fighting units were generally expected to evacuate their own casualties through a regimental aid post. Stretcher-bearers, usually chosen from the regimental band, struggled through muddy trenches to deliver casualties to a harassed medical officer. Men from one of three field ambulances in each division went forward to collect the wounded and deliver them to the division's casualty clearing station (CCS). Motor ambulances or light railways evacuated serious casualties; others might remain for surgery, treatment, and, in quiet times, a full recovery. Behind the lines, patients were directed to small "stationary hospitals" with two hundred beds or general hospitals with six hundred beds.[12]

As in other respects, the British Army was marvellously well prepared in 1914 – for another Boer War. Mass casualties soon led to a doubling of hospital size and a blurring of the distinction between general and stationary units. The CCS – as far forward as nursing sisters were allowed – gradually assumed more and more responsibility for battlefield surgery. A sharp professional debate continued through much of the war over whether the ablest surgeons should be close to the battle, where they might be killed, or remain at general hospitals, where they could repair the damage of inexperienced colleagues and do intricate, time-consuming operations.[13]

Jones had no leisure for such arguments. As the CEF expanded to four divisions by the autumn of 1916, he had to provide them with adequately trained and equipped medical units. Grim experience taught that a division in the field would suffer, on average, twenty thousand casualties a year, but they would come in alternating floods and trickles. Between the Canadian Corps' eight thousand casualties at Mont Sorrel in June 1916 and the twenty-four thousand in September and October, only a few hundred a month made their painful way back through the evacuation system. Frugal, like most peacetime soldiers, Jones saw no point in providing all the hospitals the CAMC would need in a crisis. It was far wiser to pool Canadian and British resources. Imperial-minded Canadians, including Sir George Perley, the acting Canadian high commissioner in London, entirely agreed. How better to deepen the ties of Empire than by humanitarian collaboration?[14]

By the same token, the CAMC's hospitals were shared in the common cause. In 1915 Jones bowed to a British plea to send three of his hospitals to the Mediterranean. There were no Canadian casualties, but there was a host of British and Australian sick and wounded. British gratitude was inadequate compensation for the miseries of climate, malaria, and dysentery that afflicted the CAMC personnel, or for shortages of every necessity.[15] Two other hospitals, recruited in French Canada, had a happier destiny; they were located outside Paris to serve the French army. Eight other hospitals were located on the British lines of communication, and still more were located in England. Additional special hospitals served orthopaedic, eye and ear, and mental cases. Two hospitals for venereal-disease sufferers did not have nursing sisters; two others, at Hyde Park and the Petrograd Hotel, were reserved for officers and certainly did have nursing care. After 1916 a number of convalescent hospitals were created.[16]

Among the ancillaries of the medical organization was a Canadian Army Dental Corps, created early in 1915 to ensure that soldiers could chew their army rations. Dental expertise expanded to include facial surgery, the special challenge of trench mouth, and, for those who had them, the repair of bridges and other appliances, at their owners' expense. Tucked into the original Canadian contingent was a tiny Canadian Army Hydrological Corps, a mobile laboratory under Colonel G.G. Nasmith. Its members, soon transferred to the CAMC, added significantly to Canada's medical reputation by detecting the organism that caused trench mouth and the carrier of trench fever.[17]

Understandably, the CAMC's focus was overseas. In 1914 the departure of experienced senior officers left a mere major to oversee medical arrangements in Canada. Inundated by the problems of recruiting officers and men for his corps, meeting the medical needs of a proliferation of CEF units, and enduring the snubs of his military superiors, there was much that Major J.L. Potter could not hope to accomplish. What could he do, for example, about the hundreds of doctors authorized to pass recruits as fit for service? Patriotic volunteers – and their colonels – protested at being rejected for some trifling disability. As the search for recruits grew desperate in 1916, even official standards plummeted. By the fall of 1916 up to a fifth of the Canadian soldiers arriving in England were unfit for service. Many of them never would be. Would-be soldiers arrived with missing feet, fingers, and in at least one case a completely missing forearm. Some had ulcerous open sores, and too many tested positive for tuberculosis. One eighty-nine-year old patriot from Guelph suffered from "advanced senile dementia." Many more remained in Canada as medical burdens. A third of the CEF's tuberculosis cases never got overseas; very few got close enough to poison gas to make a legitimate pension claim.[18] The blame for inadequate medical screening of recruits fell on Potter and his local physicians.

Unfit recruits were more than a nuisance. Each of them, certified fit on enlistment, posed an immediate problem of medical treatment and a potential claim on the military pension system. In 1915, when the civilian-run Military Hospitals Commission (MHC) was established to deal with returning wounded, its first and most pressing task was to look after soldiers who had never left Canada. MHC officials scrambled for hospital and sanatorium accommodation and eventually developed the commission's own facilities. Staffed by civilian physicians and by militia doctors reluctant to abandon their civilian practices, the MHC's hospitals and convalescent homes remained outside army jurisdiction until 1918. In 1915 and 1916 most CAMC officers were too busy to care.[19]

3. BATTLEFIELD SURGERY

An image of heroic humanitarianism, personified by the unassuming Scrimger or the CAMC's second VC winner, Captain B.S. Hutcheson, was a valuable asset in a war that seemed to contemporaries to strain for new depths of inhumanity. If Canadians had known more about battlefield surgery, they might not have been reassured.

Little in their training or peacetime experience prepared doctors for the casualties of trench warfare. Even in South Africa most bullet wounds healed quickly in the dry air, and shell casualties were rare. In France and Franders 28 per cent of wound were caused by bullets. High-velocity slugs shattered bones and turned flesh to pulp. Ricochets tore gaping wounds. Steel helmets, introduced in 1916, cut losses but added to the horrible consequences of a sniper's bullet through the skull. Machine guns usually caused multiple wounds, five or ten of them in a single body. Shell and grenade fragments caused almost all the rest of the wounds. Chunks of white-hot metal severed limbs, shattered faces, and left huge gaping holes, and the victims still arrived alive at aid posts and dressing stations. Lieutenant-Colonel W.L. Watts recalled the stream of Canadian wounded at Ypres: "Legs, feet, hands missing; bleeding of stumps controlled by rough field tourniquets; large portions of the abdominal walls shot away; faces horribly mutilated; bones shattered to pieces; holes that you could put your clenched fist into, filled with dirt, mud, bits of equipment and clothing, until it all becomes like a hideous nightmare."[20]

The fate of the wounded was determined by an increasingly formal process of sorting – discreetly camouflaged by the French word *triage*. Soldiers wounded during an attack or a night patrol waited in hope that someone would find them. A few survived days in no-man's land; most entered medical statistics as killed in action. Stretcher-bearers inevitably assessed the chances of dragging wounded to safety against their own fear and exhaustion, but an amazing number persisted. The luckiest wounded were those who could somehow make their own way back. By common testimony, whatever the circumstances, a wound was justification for any soldier to drop his weapon and kit and, if he could, head back. Soldiers dreamed and talked of "a Blighty," the wound that would rescue them, perhaps for the duration of the war, from the horror of the trenches. To die of wounds was to come close to the prize and then be robbed. [21]

British statistics indicated that 7 per cent of wounded soldiers died at aid posts and dressing stations and 16 per cent at clearing stations, where triage in its most obvious form segregated the hopeless cases and left them, if possible sedated and nursed, for the inevitable end. Men with stomach wounds had less than a 30 per cent chance of survival. Of 144,608 Canadian wounded who lived, only 5,233 men survived injuries to the chest, abdomen, or pelvis, compared to 22,284 who lived through wounds to the head or neck. Penetration of the pleura and the major veins and arteries by bullet or shell fragment almost certainly guaranteed that a soldier would not even be evacuated for medical attention, although a few astonishing recoveries were recorded. A fractured femur generated hypovolemic shock, leading to coma and death, usually because a wounded man had to be transported a considerable distance down winding trenches, bumping and grinding along the way. Suitable splints were devised, advertised in the medical press but almost never available when and where needed. Dressing stations applied various versions of *réchauffement* with heaters and blankets to save such cases. Blood transfusions were sometimes attempted, but blood typing was still hit or miss. [22]

For battlefield surgeons, infection was the worst enemy. Wounds in the abdomen and perineum posed a familiar problem, with potential for massive haemorrhaging and contamination from the body's own wastes and bacteria. However, military surgeons were also acutely aware of the intrusions of the battlefield. Soldiers fought amid rotting corpses, rats, germ-infested Flanders mud, and their own faeces. Fragments of uniform and equipment and local filth packed open wounds. Gas gangrene, proof against ordinary antisepsis, generated a foul anaerobic gas that literally exploded cells to produce a revolting smell, monstrous swelling, and an early, agonizing death. Medical manuals, preaching natural healing, were useless. The French discovered that gas gangrene could be controlled only by radical debridement of the wound and irrigation by a solution of sodium hypochlorite. Surgeons in England, far removed from the problem, poured scorn on such brutal methods, but for the time they worked. A typical operation turned a tiny infected wound from a jagged shell fragment into a hole two to three inches wide, six inches long, and penetrating a soldier's thigh. Constant nursing to manage the system of tubes and pumps and the painful twice-daily changing of "plugs" followed for months.[23]

In popular imagery, war wounded were usually amputees, blind, or, if relevance were sought, someone "gassed at Ypres." In practice in the CEF, out of 95,160 wounds to arms or legs, only 2,780 led to amputation. Far more lost legs than arms, partly because the latter could reach help on their own before infection set in. While 178 soldiers were discharged from the CEF as blind, fewer than half lost their sight because of wounds. Poison-gas casualties were far more common. No separate count was kept of men who died from poison gas, but 11,356 Canadians were treated in hospital. Chlorine certainly killed hundreds of men in 1915, partly because medical expertise offered casualties nothing better than bleeding or fresh air. On the whole, gas tactics favoured disablement over death, less from humanitarian motives than because of the added burden of care imposed on the enemy. Mustard gas, a powerful vesicant introduced in the summer of 1917, blistered the skin and, if inhaled, destroyed the lining of the bronchia, leading to a hideous though infrequent death. More commonly the gas burned the body wherever it was moist, producing total albeit temporary disablement and widespread fear – exactly as the opposite side would wish.[24]

Battlefield surgery was the heroic role of military medicine, a struggle against the savagery of war waged by gallant doctors in appalling circumstances. Yet the substantial triumphs of military medicine lay in prevention, not cure. A wounded soldier was a personal tragedy. A soldier with a contagious disease was a mobile machine gun, and immunization was the best available armour. Prevention also protected morale. If army doctors could do little about the ravages of poison gas, they could prevent them. Within days of the German gas attack at Ypres, soldiers were issued their first primitive flannel helmets. By 1916 it was an offence for a soldier to be without his box respirator. Certainly it was awkward to live or fight in gas masks, and gas attacks were designed to cause acute inconvenience as much as casualties. Gun crews, sweating and straining to deliver their salvoes, were a common target for a few gas shells. Those who neglected their own protection faced the serious charge of causing a "self-inflicted wound."[25]

4. MEDICINE AND HYGIENE

In some ways the army regarded most sickness as self-imposed. Through recorded history, sick soldiers had never enjoyed much sympathy from generals or doctors. Old-timers were presumed to be "swinging the lead"; younger sufferers lacked character. When the Japanese demonstrated in their war with Russia that careful hygiene could cut their casualties from sickness to a quarter of those killed in action, the British army found itself with a scientific basis for its prejudices. Canadians were ready converts. The urban public-health movement provided experts for the CEF's sanitary sections. A Canadian, Colonel J.A. Amyot of the University of Toronto, rose to be field-hygiene adviser to the British First Army. A Canadian textbook illustrating apparatus to purify water and guarantee germ-free latrines became a manual for the British army. Amyot and another Canadian officer, Major Harold Orr, devised the first practical device to sterilize uniforms and eliminate the pervasive louse.[26]

If experts could provide the knowledge, army discipline was the stern right hand of medical wisdom. Trench foot, an acute circulatory disease akin to frostbite, threatened to cripple the British army in the first winter of the war. Prevention depended on frequent changes of socks and rubbing the feet with whale-oil. Orders were issued, and officers lost their commands if trench foot reappeared in their units. Trench mouth, a gingival infection, was similarly controlled by strick oral hygiene and regular inspection by army dentists. The negligent were punished.[27]

Sanitary and military regulations could only modify some effects of the appalling living conditions in the trenches. Doctors, for example, seem to have exercised little influence on the rations served in the trenches, with the emphasis on bully beef, biscuits, tea, and synthetic jam and a lack of even the fresh vegetables included in the official scale. Skin conditions, notably scabies or the "seven-year itch," led to a quarter of all hospital admissions in the Canadian Corps in 1916. Patients were treated with sulphur ointment and sulphur baths administered at rest centres near the CCS. Trench fever, with symptoms of aching, vomiting, and diarrhoea, was endemic through much of the war. The British discreetly titled it "PUO," or "pyrexia of unknown origin," and took it for granted until 1918, when a Canadian, Captain A.C. Rankin, helped define the vector as the common flea. The Americans promptly eliminated the disease and the British followed suit. It had cost the Canadians 17,122 cases and 14 deaths.[28]

No wartime medical problem caused more controversy and concern than venereal disease. None received less sympathy. It was, Macphail curtly noted, "the least difficult of all self-inflicted wounds to inflict." The 66,083 cases in the CEF far outnumbered the 45,460 influenza cases and represented an epidemic that could not be concealed. Since it began as soon as the first Canadians reached England, moral nationalists blamed the evil of the Old World. More detached experts noted that syphilis and gonorrhoea were well known in Canada and that CEF rates, which exceeded even those of Australians, were easily attributed to high pay and remoteness from home. By 1916 a deepening manpower crisis compelled the CEF to retain its "venereals" and treat them in two special hospitals. Salvarsan, an arsenical with alarming side-effects, was the major weapon. The fact that treatment with the so-called "magic bullet" could sometimes also be exceedingly painful made it especially appropriate in a treatment program designed to be punitive and cautionary. VD sufferers were segregated; their pay was stopped, and any subsequent pension claims were often denied because syphilitic symptoms were so varied.[29]

As elsewhere, prevention was clearly better than the cure. The CEF sponsored posters and lectures and even contemplated a film until chaplains protested that it would have at least to hint at immorality. Regimental medical officers were required to inspect their soldiers' private parts at regular intervals to detect the serious offence of concealing the disease.

CAMC officers generally weighed the medical problem more heavily than moral indignation and, by 1916, began distributing prophylactic packets with a tube of calomel ointment and some potassium permanganate, which soldiers were expected to apply after intercourse. British official disapproval stopped the practice for a time, but by 1918 the Canadians had teamed up with the Australians and New Zealanders to establish treatment centres labelled "blue-light depots," where men were expected to administer prophylaxsis under supervision. By appearing to treat disease in its earliest stages rather than offering protection to the immoral, army doctors hoped to avert moral indignation from both British and Canadian public opinion. Condoms were not contemplated.[30]

Empowered by their wartime experience, some army doctors returned to civilian life persuaded that a combination of science and discipline could create a healthy post-war world. Typical among them was Captain Gordon Bates, who moved from running an anti-VD campaign for the CAMC to become secretary of the Canadian National Council for Combating Venereal Disease. It was a start to a crusading career.[31]

The war may have taught Canadian medical officers little about modern curative medicine, but it provided thousands of young practitioners with a thorough exposure to public health and hygiene. Unit medical officers, often junior members of the CAMC hierarchy, were responsible for the sanitary conditions of their battalion as well as for managing the suspect malingerers on morning sick parade. Since medical education seldom gave much grounding in practical public hygiene, CAMC officers learned on the job. The war also forced Canadians to face the full dimensions of such social-medical problems as tuberculosis and venereal disease. The shocking extent of both sets of diseases could no longer be ignored by the comfortable middle class. Wartime expansion of sanitaria to meet the needs of the CAMC and the MHC helped to transform tuberculosis treatment from a charitable to a state concern. Fear that returning soldiers would bring an epidemic of venereal diseases to Canada helped to persuade Ottawa to establish a Department of Health, while between 1917 and 1929 all provinces imposed some form of compulsory treatment.[32]

5. "SHELL SHOCK"

In pre-war Canada psychiatry was already very largely part of state medicine. Huge provincial asylums warehoused patients for whom no real cure was expected. Orthodox opinion linked mental disturbances to organic causes and usually to heredity. Few ambitious physicians were drawn to a field that offered uncongenial patients, meagre therapeutic possibilities, and a modest government salary.[33]

The advent of war changed nothing. The CAMC felt no need to add 'alienists" to its professional ranks. Manly courage was taken for granted among those who composed the CEF; cowardice or desertion in the face of the enemy was punished by death. Exhaustion could be cured by a day's rest or a good night's sleep. Among some front-line medical officers, experience of trench warfare modified such complacent conclusions. Captain R.J. Manion, who served with the French and the Canadians, recalled the tragic transformation of hitherto excellent soldiers: "He trembles violently, his heart may be disordered in rhythm, he has a terrified air, the slightest noise makes him jump and even occasionally run at top speed to a supposed place of safety."[34]

Early in the war medical officers were forced to deal with soldiers displaying inexplicable paralyses, mutism, deafness, and uncontrollable crying. Faith in somatic theory led doctors to find an analogy in soldiers found dead without a scratch after a nearby shellburst. The condition was labelled "shell shock"; sufferers were evacuated from battle, frequently discharged, and offered food, rest, and much sympathy. Notably, they were rarely cured. Cases returned to Canada were housed at a special hospital in Cobourg; it was intolerable that suffering heroes should come in contact with mere lunatics.[35]

Even if it had been successful, neither generals nor doctors could long have tolerated such treatment. Who would have been left to man the trenches? By late 1916 British authorities banned the term "shell shock." Cases were labelled NYD(N), or "not yet diagnosed (nervous)." As such, they were not sick or wounded. The medical profession borrowed a more detailed typology from peacetime psychiatry. Neurasthenia – exhaustion of the nervous system – explained some cases, most commonly those of officers. The cure was rest and recreation, sometimes, as with the poet Wilfred Owen, in the north of Scotland, sometimes in the south of France. An alternative diagnosis was hysteria, commonly found before the war in women confined to charity wards. Shell shock, insisted the Canadian medical historian Sir Andrew Macphail, was no more than "a manifestation of childishness and femininity." Mutism, a common sympton, was no more, suggested Sir Frederick Mott, than a private soldier's wilful evasion of his duty of silent obedience.[36]

From the diagnosis came the treatment. Lewis Yealland had returned from Canada just before the war to become resident physician at the famous Queen's Square Hospital in London. His "Black Chamber" soon became famous for its cures. Patients, suitably briefed, were strapped to a table and subjected to high-voltage electricity. One stubborn case took several hours with the "electric brush" before he could speak clearly and volubly. Six other cases of mutism were cured in half an hour, two of them merely by being shown the instruments. Yealland took pains: "You have not recovered yet," he warned a patient; "your laugh is most offensive to me." It was fixed in five minutes. A Canadian special hospital at Ramsgate borrowed Yealland's technique and claimed a 70 per cent success rate.[37]

The British and Canadians were not alone in using shock therapy; the French made even more lavish claims for their version of *torpillage*. Still, the treatment raised questions. Were doctors entitled to inflict pain for such a purpose? Yes, replied the British psychiatrist William Bailey, "in the special circumstances of a war for civilization." The agony of shock therapy, "as severe as anything we know," confessed a practitioner, restored pride and a sense of worth in men who felt disgraced by cowardice. "It gives the man the excuse to tell his comrades he was received some powerful treatment," explained Lieutenant-Colonel C.K. Russell, who commanded the Ramsgate Hospital: "He can thus save his face."[38]

In practice, even such heroic remedies failed to satisfy the army. Most British and Canadian divisions used rest camps to save soldiers who seemed to be on the edge of what, in a later war, would be called "battle fatigue." Other divisions insisted on ignoring the problem. Sir Archibald Macdonell insisted that his First Division would not acknowledge shell shock. As a result, he boasted, it did not exist. Numbers of soldiers from all four Canadian divisions found another way out. Of twenty-five Canadian soldiers executed in France, twenty-two were sentenced for desertion and one for cowardice. Many others, sentenced to death for similar behaviour, were saved by commutation. War memoirs occasionally recall their misery, though rarely with much sympathy. The ethos of the time had to insist on the universal presence of "manly virtues" among Canadian soldiers and to assume that shortcomings were individual failures of character. Officers, judged by their own equals in status and social background, fared better than men in the ranks. Among officers cashiered and imprisoned for cowardice, Lieutenant F.M. Leader, had not, as his former colonel and wife insisted, "fallen among friends" when he joined a battalion in France.[39]

The CAMC, for all its statistics, kept no record of the numbers who were diagnosed as suffering from shell shock, though about ten thousand soldiers were treated or discharged for psychiatric reasons – about half being labelled "nervous." Since the British total of eighty thousand is plainly arbitrary and almost certainly understated, the lack of Canadian figures may be only relative. Psychiatry did not add much in wartime to its dismal reputation. Although the methods of Queen's Square did not travel back to Canada, neuropsychiatric victims were denied pensions until at least 1925 on the argument that men who had avoided danger must have no financial excuse for avoiding work.[40]

Public opinion eventually forced Ottawa to recognize its responsibility for men damaged in mind as well as in body. The only two purpose-built veterans' hospitals erected after the war, Westminster in London and Ste-Anne de Bellevue in Montreal, were designed for the CEF's neuropsychiatric cases. By 1928 such cases formed a quarter of all disabled veterans; by the eve of the Second World War they were close to half. Yet so stagnant was the progress of military psychiatry that Colonel Russell could offer his heirs in the new conflict nothing better than the electric brush "as a ready means of cleaning up the condition."[41]

6. PERSONALITIES AND POLITICS

Since medical care had largely been limited to those who could afford it, pre-war Canada had more doctors than could make a comfortable living. Even when the CAMC had begun its rapid expansion, it was possible to make four hundred practitioners available to the hard-pressed British. Only by 1916, when the full dimensions of the war became apparent, did Canadians begin to recognize a doctor shortage. Medical schools accelerated and abbreviated their courses, and medical students who had enlisted as orderlies in university-based hospital units were sent back to Canada to complete a hurried training.[42]

Doctors who joined the CEF entered a world very different from civilian practice, or even from the peacetime militia. Professional competence varied enormously; so did qualifications. The CAMC included recent graduates of McGill or Toronto, physicians and surgeons with well-earned international reputations, and elderly practitioners who had qualified at the Manitoba Medical College in the 1870s. All ranked at least as captains, with seniority over almost all nurses but with no right to command combatant troops other than their patients. Yet doctors were to be disciplinarians, reporting such crimes as self-inflicted wounds and remembering that the army's need for men outranked concern for patient welfare. These were hard lessons for any civilians in uniform to learn. Some doctors, like the famous Colonel McCrae, had long thought of themselves as soldiers; others had to adapt.[43]

Expanded and improvised as it was, the CAMC worked best in France, where such conditions were understood. Despite the hardships and dangers of working close to the trenches, morale was generally highest among men who knew the value of their work. Working closely with the Royal Army Medical Corps (RAMC) allowed the Canadians to adopt or adapt British examples. The chief resentment, as in all field armies, was with officers at the base. "No reward comes to a man who does his work faithfully," complained Macphail in May of 1916 when he served with a field ambulance in France, "Appointments and promotions are made from London, without any regard to service or seniority in the Field. Men arrive from Canada as Majors and Colonels who had not even joined when we left."[44]

Such complaints are traditional in armies. In England and in Canada, far from battle, the CAMC was on its own. The chaos inevitable in an improvised army, aggravated by the croneyism of Sir Sam Hughes, the minister of Militia, extended to the medical services. Discipline and regulations were haphazardly enforced, adding to the sense of injustice and discontent. Between the rushes of casualties, hospital staffs were frequently underemployed and prey to intrigues about promotion, transfers, and leave. Wives often joined their husbands in England and created their own network. The more successful practitioners in civil life found a captain's pay (three dollars a day) and status a humiliation. Resentment focused on General Jones, whom the waspish Macphail dismissed as "a stupid, heavy-witted man" who physically resembled no one so much as the hated German Kaiser. Jones's chosen subordinates, permanent-force officers trying to impose army ways on civilian professionals, were no better loved.[45]

Discontented doctors had plenty of criticisms. Why had Jones squandered three of the best Canadian hospitals on the Mediterranean, where conditions were abominable? Why had he not created enough hospitals so that Canadian sick and wounded need not be scattered among hundreds of British hospitals, often under the amateurish nursing care of the Voluntary Aid Detachments (VAD)? Additional Canadian institutions would have meant opportunities and promotions for CAMC officers and better control of Canadian manpower. Was Jones doing all that he could to solve the increasingly desperate manpower shortage that faced the CEF by mid-1916? And who but senior officers of the CAMC could be blamed for increasing numbers of unfit and unsuitable recruits arriving from Canada? In Canada medical corps officers came increasingly to recent the spreading authority of the Military Hospitals Commission and its habit of putting ex-combatant officers in charge of its convalescent homes and hospitals in order to enforce discipline. What else could one expect from an organization run by civilians, whose medical superintendent, Colonel Alfred Thompson, was best known as a mining speculator and MP for the Yukon?[46]

In the summer of 1916, forced to reform his embattled department, Sir Sam Hughes announced sweeping investigations of the medical services in Canada and overseas. The overseas inquiry was assigned to Colonel Herbert A. Bruce, the founder of the Wellesley Hospital and a briskly efficient Toronto surgeon. Whether Hughes knew or cared, Bruce was a man with a score to settle. An earlier brief period of service in France had ended with charges that he had betrayed military secrets to the press and purloined public property – to wit, X-ray plates Bruce had taken home to use in medical lectures.[47] His accuser, General Jones, would now be judged. Bruce's verdict was predictable; his sweeping indictment of the CAMC was not. A *pro forma* assertion that medical officers and nursing sisters were doing work "beyond all praise" was followed by detailed condemnation. Under Jones the medical corps had encouraged unqualified surgeons to hone their art on Canadian boys. Medical officers included incompetents, alcoholics, and outright "drug fiends." An unhealthy hint of scandal surrounded the Duchess of Connaught's Red Cross Hospital at Taplow, a major Canadian establishment where senior medical officers were suspected of abusing their perquisites for pleasure or profit. British hospitals, where most Canadians recuperated, were little better than marriage bureaus for untrained VAD nurses. Canadians, Bruce reported, had begged him for a transfer to their own hospitals.[48]

Even worse than the administrative bungling Bruce claimed to have discovered was the fact that eminent practitioners like himself had to place their reputations in the hands of doctors whose claim to rank was pre-war service in the permanent force. It was well known, Bruce later claimed, "that it is not necessarily the ablest physician or surgeon who is given the premier position in a military organization. In fact one can assert without exaggeration that frequently the reverse is the case." The answer, Bruce reported, would be a board of consultants whose advice would be binding on military authorities. Since any senior officer might be scientifically backward, "it would be nothing short of criminal that he be given autocratic powers that would enable him to nullify the decisions of a body of experts."[49]

Sir Sam Hughes was delighted by a report that played to his own brash nationalism and to his contempt for military professionals. Jones was fired and replaced by Colonel Bruce. Hardly was the deed done than Hughes himself was dismissed by an exasperated prime minister. The newly created Ministry of the Overseas Military Forces of Canada inherited the medical imbroglio. Its new minister, Sir George Perley, later confessed that he would never have accepted the job had he known the difficulties. Some of them he and Lady Perley had aggravated by their strong backing of General Jones, but they were not alone. Bruce's arrogance and his sweeping charges made even Macphail a defender of the Jones regime. Sir William Osler, the great Canadian physician and a consultant to the CAMC, resigned in fury when Bruce was appointed. Other medical officers shared his indignation.[50]

Perley did what he could. A prominent British surgeon-general, Sir William Babtie, headed a committee of Canadian medical officers, including a couple of Bruce partisans, to review the Bruce report. Its tone and criticisms were rejected; its reforms were largely implemented. Canadian hospitals were brought back from Salonika as part of a vastly expanded network of institutions. Convalescent beds were increased tenfold to well over seven thousand. Under Perley military regulations largely supplanted personal and political influence. Jones, briefly restored, was soon replaced by Major-General G.L. Foster, another Nova Scotia–born permanent force officer who had won respect for managing the medical services of the Canadian

Corps in France. Even Bruce's proposal for a medical board and surgical consultants was belatedly adopted late in 1918, though Canadian hospitals had been inspected by eminent British specialists.[51]

Perley's arrangements did not end intrigue or dissatisfaction. CAMC files are thick with disputes, complaints, and symptoms of injured dignity. Bruce and his partisans continued a vendetta that soon shifted its targets to Perley, Foster, and other sources of their humiliation. The government had its own answer. Macphail won promotion and a knighthood for his zeal in defending the CAMC and its commanders in a campaign that extended to his post-war authorship of the official history of the CEF's medical services. Perhaps preserving public confidence in wartime medical arrangements was a war-winning service. Another prominent critic, Brigadier-General Charles Smart, was silenced by reminders that he had spent most of his brief overseas service in one of the VAD hospitals in the south of France. There may also have been discreet reminders that he had spent time as a patient in one of the CAMC's psychiatric wards in Ste-Anne de Bellevue.[52]

7 · REHABILITATION

In Canada, Bruce's counterpart was a youthful Toronto gynaecologist and CAMC pioneer, Colonel Frederick Marlow. More sympathetic to wartime growing pains, Marlow's chief concern was to overthrow the authority of the Military Hospitals Commission and end the scandal of unfit recruits. The latter was achieved by centralizing medical examinations in major centres, where X-ray machines and other diagnostic equipment could be collected. By 1918, when the CAMC was more involved in compelling conscripts to serve than in rejecting unsuitable volunteers, the machinery was working much more smoothly.[53] The battle with the MHC caused more trouble. Pointing to the MHC's failures only embarrassed and angered its political chiefs. Marlow's argument that "putting invalid soldiers under civilian control broke the Geneva Convention" left a parliamentary committee skeptical. Senator Sir James Lougheed easily defeated Colonel Marlow, but he finally lost his own year-long battle for control of military hospitals in Canada. In March 1918 the MHC was dissolved and most of its institutions were transferred to the Militia Department.[54]

The CAMC, however, had won only a token triumph. Its new beds were a wasting asset. As the end of the war approached, its ablest doctors thought only of an early return to their civilian practices.

When the 1918 influenza epidemic proved unexpectedly fatal to scores of young men in military hospitals, the CAMC took the blame. Operating hospitals close to unfettered public opinion was uncomfortable. "The grumbler, the malingerer and the neurotic," complained Macphail, "never failed to find an audience equally neurotic."[55] The CAMC's defence of its administration – that it had cut costs and resisted pressure for needless expansion – somehow won fewer friends than the authorities hoped.

For all its internal turmoil and external failings, the CAMC had legitimately earned the respect of contemporary Canadians. Heroism and self-sacrifice in humanitarian service continued through the war to give army doctors and nurses a special aura. The generalized horror of war took on a Canadian specificity when Canadian general hospitals were bombed in May 1918 and when the hospital ship *Llandovery Castle* was torpedoed and its few lifeboats shelled. Every nursing sister aboard was drowned.

Yet the fundamental purpose of military medicine was not self-sacrifice but the conservation of manpower for a military purpose. The needs of a citizen army forced the CAMC to settle policy issues that still trouble the managers of state-run medical systems. According to the cautious words of its Board of Consultants, "The policy and object kept steadily in view has been to secure and provide economically, but not parsimoniously, for the invalid soldier the best possible care and treatment upon the most modern lines, ... so as to fit him in the speediest way for return to duty or, where that is impossible, for his discharge at the earliest possible moment after treatment has attained finality, and the highest possible fitness [been] secured."[56]

What was possible, of course, depended on the doctor, the invalid, and the state of knowledge. What was certain was that public opinion and the Canadian economy could not accept the traditional detritus of a great war – throngs of sick, disabled veterans subsisting on meagre pensions and charity. A little experience persuaded medical authorities that more than kindness was needed to restore disabled soldiers to self-sufficiency. There was also an edge of resentment that former labourers should live in idleness. Invalids, warned the CAMC's Colonel Alexander Primrose, "have become accustomed to having everything done for them, they lose all ambition and have no desire to help themselves."[57] The MHC's rehabilitation policy, developed as early as the summer of 1915 by its secretary, Ernest Scammell, was designed to persuade veterans to fend for themselves. Those who could return to old jobs had no further claim on the state; those who had lost their trade through sickness or wounds must be retrained as rapidly as possible to a corresponding level of skill.[58]

The French, with their huge casualty toll, showed Canadians what could be done to restore and train the maimed survivors. Major J.L. Todd, sidelined for pension duties, reported enthusiastically on French achievements. In Canada, Scammell proved an eager disciple. The MHC also learned that even the bedridden could be coerced into old work disciplines through "ward occupations" and "curative workshops." Only when discharged from treatment could ex-soldiers learn new trades – ideally on the job. In turn the MHC and its successor, the Department of Soldiers' Civil Re-establishment (DSCR), had to persuade employers that the disabled could be valuable workers. Military hospitals set an example. Blinded soldiers were employed as masseurs. Amputees went to work in the MHC's artificial-limb factory in Toronto. The CAMC's only female amputee was employed as a social worker for tubercular veterans. The sole quadrilateral amputee, Private "Curly" Christian, was found a job as a billiard marker.[59]

The military pension system, devised in 1916 by Major Todd, attempted to reinforce the principles of rehabilitation. Based on French and British experience and a fear of the American pension evil, Canadian pensions were generous on paper but tight-fisted in practice. Medical boards were expected to define a soldier's disabilities precisely. Medical examiners, working from the reports, assessed disability as a fraction of what might be expected from an unskilled labourer and assigned the appropriate pension. Pre-enlistment disabilities, whenever discernible, were deducted. Of seventy thousand disability pensions awarded by 1920, fewer than five thousand recognized full or near-full disability, while half were for 20 per cent or less.[60] Returned soldiers had plenty of incentive to find work. In the postwar book of 1919, when it was both patriotic and profitable to hire returned soldiers, they could and did find jobs; in the depression of 1920–21, many found themselves unemployed. Memories, as both Scammell and Todd had warned, were short.[61]

8.   BRAVE NEW WORLD

Like other veterans, doctors and nursing sisters came home to a Canada more eager to welcome than to re-employ them. Both professions had grown substantially during the war years; nursing had almost doubled. Military hospitals, shrinking as fast as the war receded, could employ only a few hundred nurses and few doctors.

Not all nurses could follow the traditional exit. "Scores of our nurses are marrying every week," wrote thrity-five-year-old Frances Upton to her father, "but not the old ones like myself who have tired themselves out with hard work."[62] Among doctors, prominent specialists faced the least difficulty re-establishing themselves. Their youngest colleagues, such as Fred Banting, needed refresher courses to complete an abbreviated wartime training. Middle-aged physicians faced the hardest prospect: rebuilding a practice at a time when contemporaries were close to their maximum earning power. Medical associations and journals were full of schemes to redistribute patients, but, as Colonel E.J. Williams rapidly concluded, "the feasibility of them all is doubtful in the extreme."[63]

An alternative, urged even in the *Canadian Medical Association Journal*, was adoption of some form of Britain's pre-war health-insurance scheme. The war, claimed Colonel J.L. Biggar, had demonstrated that Canadians were unfit; it also showed how to cure the problem. "A State medical system is today providing treatment for many thousands of ex-service men discharged, disabled or diseased, to civil life."[64] A Vancouver doctor proposed a contract plan, with the poor enabled at last to seek expert medical opinion. How better, he argued, to find employment for a hundred colleagues returning from the war. Wartime experience and a willingness to contemplate a brave new post-war world made reform seem easy. Major Todd predicted to an American audience in November 1918 that "the fact that former sailors and soldiers and their families are protected against risks of death, accident and ill-health will inevitably lead towards the extension of social, health and life insurance to all citizens."[65]

The inevitable would take a long time. The mood of radical innovation that Todd had detected during the last years of the war was exhausted after the armistice. Nostalgia replaced expectation. Returning soldiers proved on the whole to be a conservative influence as they asserted their stake in a society they had helped to defend. Having experienced the collectivism of military life and a particularly oppressive form of socialized medicine, they were awkward allies for those who would return to the old individualism. Veterans' hospitals gradually closed during the 1920s, leaving only a few large establishments such as Toronto's Christie Street and Calgary's Colonel Belcher Hospital, and the psychiatric hospitals outside London and Montreal. Free medical care, nervously extended to all returned soldiers for a year after the war, was rigorously restricted thereafter to disabled pensioners suffering permanent injury or recurring sickness. The medical profession soon forgot its brief flirtation with state-run health systems – at least until the Depression, when physicians again ran short of private income.[66] Doctors, like other Canadians, gradually heeded the advice of Colonel Clarence Starr, a renowned Toronto orthopaedic surgeon, who declared on his return: "The sooner we in Canada get away from military titles and everything connected with the war, the better it will be for the country and the average citizen."[67]

Historians could not be as forgetful. Had the war been a catalyst for medical innovation or a tremendous distraction? Had the disciplined team effort created by military medicine produced a sharing of advances or a stultification of initiative? Had the massive invasion from North America brought more than hookworm to Europe – or athlete's foot to Canada and the United States? "The great, outstanding feature of the War," wrote McGill's Dr George Adami in 1920, "has been the triumph of preventive medicine."[68] Admittedly, inoculation, vaccination, and germ theory were all established before 1914, but wartime experience in controlling contagion gave doctors and the public a faith in prevention they had never had before. Vaccination was 125 years old, but it had seemed a bold measure in 1914 to enforce it on the CEF. By 1915 immunization was automatic at every stage of a soldier's move to the front.[69]

Compared to medicine, surgical advances seemed less dramatic and relevant to civilian practice. Gas gangrene was an unlikely outcome of a peacetime operation. Civilian physicians deplored the surgical over-specialization natural in army medical officers coping with casualties by the thousand. Returning doctors, specialized in facial mutilations or compound fractures, were hardly prepared for the variety of individualized peacetime practice. At the same time, only war could have forced the pace in reconstructive surgery or allowed practitioners of blood transfusion to improve their primitive techniques.[70]

In a far different realm, returning medical officers adapted their experience to the brand new field of industrial medicine, tackling occupational diseases, industrial hazards, and the unhygienic conditions of workplace life. Captain Bernard Wyatt, an apostle for the new specialty, reminded employers that "our great Canadian industries cannot maintain their place in the world's competition unless their employees are in good physical condition."[71]

Whether or not employers believed such a claim, wartime medicine was a powerful experiential argument for many doctors. As Robin Keirstead has pointed out, post-war addresses to medical associations bristled with military metaphors as Canadian doctors inspired each other to believe that discipline, organization, and what generals had called "the offensive spirit" could put to flight the traditional enemies of human health. Army experience with preventive medicine was a standing demonstration that society as a whole must arise against such common threats as tuberculosis and syphilis. The public, too, realized that war had its humanitarian as well as its military victories and that in both spheres only teamwork produced results.

The experience of war was a catalyst for change, but there were conservative influences to buffer the speed of the reaction. Disease remained, for most Canadians, a self-inflicted wound, whether it took the form of shell shock or pneumonia, and much of military hygiene was an attempt to apply army discipline to the control of personal habits. The memory of pre-dawn sick parades – designed to discourage the more faint-hearted malingerers – and the weekly short-arm inspections would pervade a generation's image of what "state" medicine would entail for both practitioners and patients. The post-1918 image of health insurance as a means of distributing poor patients among underemployed doctors had too much of the army in it to be welcome, even to veterans. Canadian medicine would be free to muddle along for another generation or more.[72]

NOTES

1 J.L. Todd, "The Meaning of Rehabilitation," *Annals of the American Academy of Political and Social Science* 80 (Nov. 1918): 1.

2 Sir Andrew Macphail, *Official History of the Canadian Forces in the Great War, 1914–1919: The Medical Services* (Ottawa 1925), 6, 329, and on strength of permanent force, 316; *Report of the Ministry of Overseas Military Forces of Canada, 1918* (London, nd), 394–401, on strength and disposition of the wartime CAMC. On numbers see "Canadian Army Medical Corps: Reorganization," editorial, *Canadian Medical Association Journal* 21 (1921): 964. On the Canadian medical profession see C. David Naylor, *Private Practice, Public Payment: Canadian Medicine and the Politics of Health Insurance, 1911–1966* (Montreal and Kingston: McGill's-Queen's University Press 1986), 16–26.

3 Of the wounded and injured, 34,079 were discharged from the CEF as unfit. Major Clyde R. Scott to Secretary, Board of Pension Commissioners, 29 Dec. 1927, NAC RG 24, vol. 1844, GAQ 11–11. On casualties: G.W.L. Nicholson, *Canadian Expeditionary Force, 1914–1919: The Official History of the Canadian Army in the First World War* (Ottawa: Queen's Printer 1960), 548.

4 Department of Militia and Defence, *Supplementary Report: Organization, Equipment, Despatch and Service of the Canadian Contingents During the War in South Africa, 1899–1900* (Ottawa 1901), 56–8, 104, 114, 151, 178.

5 See, for example, R.J. Manion, *Life Is an Adventure* (Toronto 1936), 157–8; Col. J.E. Squire, *Medical Hints for the Use of Medical Officers Temporarily Employed with Troops* (London 1915); Col. H.A. Bruce, "Surgical Efficiency in an Army Medical Service," *CMA Journal* 9 (1919): 988–90. These and other references in the medical literature are suggested by Robin Keirstead's "Doctors at War: The Canadian Military Medical Experience, 1914–1918," MA, Queen's 1983. His own treatment of this subject can be found on pp 27–38.

6 Typical of soldier responses to medical officers was W.R. Bird, *Ghosts Have Warm Hands*, new ed. (Toronto: Clarke-Irwin 1968), 22–3. See Dennis Winter, *Death's Men* (London: Penguin 1978).

7 Nurses, claimed an official medical historian, had a higher status in Canada than in Britain, as the profession "attracts, in general, the daughters of professional men, and those from comfortable households" had, in many cases, missed out in the marriage market. See J.G. Adami, *The War Story of the CAMC*, vol. I, *The First Contingent, 1914–1915* (London, nd), 34. See also G.W.L. Nicholson, *Canada's Nursing Sisters* (Toronto: Samuel, Stevens 1975).

8 On immunization, Keirstead, "Doctors," 143–8: Adami, *War Story*, 43. There was no general medical agreement on the efficacy of typhoid vaccine until the 1950s. See Wesley W. Spink, *Infectious Diseases: Prevention and Treatment in the Nineteenth and Twentieth Centuries* (Minneapolis: University of Minnesota Press 1978), 244. Even vaccination was controversial in 1914, 150 years after Jenner.

9 On the meningitis epidemic, Macphail, *Medical Services*, 257–9; Lt Col. J.W.S. McCullough, "Sanitation in War," *CMA Journal* 9 (1919): 787; Col. John Adami, "Medicine and the War," ibid., 891.

10 Nicholson, *CEF*, 92. On Scrimger, J.A. Swettenham, *Valiant Men: Canadian Victoria Cross and George Cross Winners* (Toronto: Hakkert/Canadian War Museum 1973), 37.

11 Adami, *War Service*, 26–7.

12 On procedures at the front, see Macphail, *Medical Services*, 129–36 or, more briefly, John Ellis, *Eye Deep in Hell: The Western Front, 1914–1918* (London: Croom Helm 1976), 108–10.

13 Macphail, *Medical Services*, 120–5; John Laffin, *Surgeons in the Field* (London: Dent 1970), 223 *et passim*. The ruthless speed of battlefield surgery and the technique of debriding led to criticism of frontline surgeons by eminent civilian surgeons working in British or Canadian hospitals in England and fed many of Bruce's attacks in 1916. Norman Bethune, a CAMC surgeon, suffered such criticism throughout his

post-war career. See H. Rocke Robertson, "Edward Archibald, the 'New Medical Science' and Norman Bethune," in Davis A.E. Shephard and Andrée Lévesque, eds., *Norman Bethune: His Times and His Legacy* (Ottawa: University of Ottawa Press 1982), 74–5.

14 Macphail, *Medical Services*, 162–5.

15 Ibid., 295–6; Nicholson, CEF, 497–8.

16 Macphail, *Medical Services*, 218, 235–7, 294; H.A. Bruce, *Report on the Canadian Army Medical Service* (London 1916), 43ff.

17 On the CADC: *Report of the OMBC, 1918*, 405–7.

18 Ibid., 157–61. See Keirstead, "Doctors at War," 23–6. On the evidence: Maj. W.F. Kemp to Adjutant-General, CEF, 31 Oct. 1916, NAC RG 9, III, vol. 90, 10–12–15; GOC Canadians to Secretary, Militia Council, 18 July 1916, RG 24, vol. 1144, HQ 54–21–51; NAC MG 30, E-3, vol. 3. On problems with tubercular recruits: Katherine McCuaig, "From Social Reform to Social Science: The Changing Role of Volunteers: The Anti-Tuberculosis Campaign, 1900–1930," *Canadian Historical Review* 61 (1980): 485–6; and on general consequences of enlisting the unfit, Desmond Morton and Glenn Wright, *Winning the Second Battle: Canadian Veterans and the Return to Civilian Life 1915–1930* (Toronto: University of Toronto Press 1987), 24–7.

19 On the MHC, ibid., 14–18 *et passim*.

20 Cited in Adami, *War Service*, 118–19. See Major Edward Archibald, "A Brief Survey of Some Experiences in the Surgery of the Present War," *CMA Journal* 6 (1916): 791.

21 Ellis, *Eye Deep*, 114; Winter, *Death's Men*, 193–4.

22 Survival rates are in Macphail, *Medical Services*, 396. On femur fractures, see ibid., 113–16; Ellis, *Eye Deep*, 111; Keirstead, "Doctors at War," 93–4.

23 For descriptions of gas gangrene and its treatment: Frederick A. Pottle, *Stretchers: The Story of a Hospital Unit on the Western Front* (New Haven 1929), 109–10, 138–9, 154–5. A vivid Canadian description by Thomas Geggie is in *Toronto Daily Star*, 27 Mar. 1917. See Major Edward Archibald, "A Brief Survey of Some Experiences in the Surgery of the Present War," *CMA Journal* 6 (1916): 791; Lt Col. G.W. Crile, "Treatment of Four Hundred and Twenty Infected Wounds under Battle Conditions," ibid. 8 (1918): 963.

24 For total amputations, see Macphail, *Medical Services*, 396–7; Royal Commission on Pensions, *Final Report* (Ottawa 1925), 51. On the blind, Canadian House of Commons, *Proceedings of the Special Committee ... to Report upon the Reception, Treatment, Care, Training and Re-education of the Wounded, Disabled and Convalescent ... 1917* (Ottawa 1918), 109–10, 559–60. On gas and the effects, Keirstead, "Doctors at War," 225–7; Macphail, *Medical Services*, 299–306. On use of bleeding,

Major G.B. Peat, "The Effects of Gassing as Seen at a Casualty Clearing Station," *CMA Journal* 8 (1918): 23.

25 On protection, Ellis, *Eye Deep*, 66; Kierstead, "Doctors at War," 225–6. On experience with respirators, see Bird, *Ghosts*, 98–9. On pension consequences for men who forgot their respirators, Morton and Wright, *Second Battle*, 159. On a soldier's experiences with gas, R.H. Roy, ed., *The Journal of Private Fraser, 1914–1918* (Vancouver: Sono Nis Press 1985), 96–7, 188–9, 277–9.

26 Macphail, *Medical Services*, 237–8, 275; McCullough, "Sanitation," 783–5, refers to the Japanese experience. On medical attitudes to the sick, see Macphail diaries, NAC MG 30 D 150, vol. 4 – for example, 28 Oct. 1916: "The wards look like the interior of the Old Brewery Mission. These men have a genius for discovering the easy place, and hospital accommodation is so enormous that they have little difficulty in gaining admission."

27 On trench foot: Macphail, *Medical Services*, 269–70; Nicholson, CEF, 126–7; Major F. McKelvey Bell, "Effects of Wet and Cold: Trench Foot," *CMA Journal* 6 (1916): 290–1. On trench mouth, Macphail, *Medical Services*, 270–1; Keirstead, "Doctors at War," 173–4.

28 Ibid., 162–8; Macphail, *Medical Services*, 237, 262–3; on the disease see Major W. Byam, Captains J.H. Carroll, J.H. Churchill, Lyn Dimond, V.E. Sorapire, R.M. Wilson, and L.L. Loyd, *Trench Fever: A Louse-Borne Disease* (London 1919).

29 On VD, see Suzann Buckley and Janice Dickin McGinniss, "Venereal Disease and Public Health Reform in Canada," *Canadian Historical Review* 63 (1982): 344ff; Janice Dickin McGinniss, "From Salvarsan to Pencillin: Medical Science and VD Control in Canada"; Wendy Mitchinson and Janice Dickin McGinnis, *Essays in the History of Canadian Medicine* (Toronto: McClelland and Stewart 1988), 126ff; Jay Cassel, *The Secret Plague: Venereal Disease in Canada 1838–1939* (Toronto: University of Toronto Press 1987), 122–44; Macphail, *Medical Services*, 29, 279.

30 On prevention, Macphail, ibid., 287–94; Cassel, *Secret Plague*, chap. 6; Lt Col. F.S. Patch, "The Military Aspect of the Venereal Disease Problem in Canada," *Canadian Journal of Public Health* 8 (1917).

31 See Captain Gordon Bates, "Venereal Disease from the Preventive Aspects," *CMA Journal* 9 (1919): 310ff; Cassel, *Secret Plague*, 171–2, 211–14.

32 Colonel G. Adami, "Medicine and the War," *CMA Journal* 10 (1920): 882ff; L.W. Harrison, "The Modern Treatment of Syphilis," ibid. 7 (1917): 31–43; McCullough, "Sanitation"; Keirstead, "Doctors at War," 174–82. On Department of Health, see Buckley and McGinniss, "Ve-

nereal Disease and Public Health," and Cassel, *Secret Plague*, 168–70 *et passim*. On arrangements to report VD cases on return to Canada, see Francis Carman, *The Return of the Troops: A Plain Account of the Demobilization of the Canadian Expeditionary Force* (Ottawa 1920), 107, 110.

33 One view of pre-war psychiatry in Canada is found in Thomas E. Brown, "Dr. Ernest Jones, Psychoanalysis and the Canadian Medical Profession," in S.E.D. Shortt, *Medicine in Canadian Society: Historical Perspectives* (Montreal: McGill-Queen's University Press 1981), 347–50.

34 R.J. Manion, *A Surgeon in Arms* (New York 1918), 163–4.

35 See Major E.H. Young, "The Care of Military Mental Patients," CMA *Journal* 9 (1919): 896 *et passim*. On Cobourg and Canadian attitudes, Morton and Wright, *Second Battle*, 27, 39.

36 Macphail's opinion is in *Medical Services*, 278. See also 276–9. A contemporary approach to typology is Captain H.P. Wright, "Suggestion for a Further Classification of Cases of So-called Shell Shock," CMA *Journal* 7 (1917): 630–3; Major C.K. Russell, "Study of Certain Psychogenetic Casualties Among Soldiers," ibid., 704–20. For a modern review see Thomas E. Brown, "Shell Shock in the Canadian Expeditionary Force, 1914–1918: Canadian Psychiatry in the Great War," in C.G. Roland, ed., *Health, Disease and Medicine: Essays in Canadian History* (Hamilton: Hannah Institute/Clarke-Irwin 1984). See also Major Norman Q. Brill, "War Neuroses," *Journal of Laboratory and Clinical Medicine* 28 (1943): 484ff.

37 Lewis R. Yealland, *Hysterical Disorders of Warfare* (London 1918), 8–23 *et passim*.

38 Keirstead, "Doctors at War," 221–6; Brown, "Shell Shock," 219–21; Lt Col. C.K. Russell, "The Nature of War Neuroses," CMA *Journal* 61 (1939): 550 for citation. See also Russell, "Psychogenetic Conditions in Soldiers: Their Aetiology, Treatment and Final Disposal," *Canadian Medical Week* (Toronto 1918), 227–37.

39 On treatment in France, Captain Edward Ryan, "A Case of Shell Shock," CMA *Journal* 6 (1916): 1095–7. On executions, Desmond Morton, "The Supreme Penalty: Canadian Deaths by Firing Squad in the First World War," *Queen's Quarterly* 79 (1972): 347–8.

40 On pension policy, see Canada House of Commons, *Proceedings of the Special Committee ... on Pension ... 1918* (Ottawa 1918), 156–8; Desmond Morton, "Resisting the Pension Evil: Bureaucracy, Democracy, and Canada's Board of Pension Commissioners, 1916–33," *Canadian Historical Review* 68 (1987): 207, 211. See minutes of meeting of 4 Sept. 1918, NAC RG 9 IIIB 2, vol. 3580, f 22–400, p 257, on board pension policy. Revision came later from the Royal Commission on Pensions in 1924; see Morton and Wright, *Second Battle*, 176.

41 Russell, "War Neuroses," 550. On interwar patient load, *Report of the Department of Soldiers' Civil Re-Establishment, 1924* (Ottawa 1926), 7; J.P. Cathcart, "The Neuro-Psychiatric Branch of the Department of Soldiers' Civil Re-establishment," *Ontario Journal of Neuro-Psychiatry* (May 1928): 44–6; Brown, "Shell Shock," 309ff.

42 On medical manpower, Keirstead, "Doctors at War," 19–22.

43 On discipline and medical officers, see ibid., 45–52. See also Squire, "*Medical Hints,*" 10–11 *et passim;* "The Canadian Medical Profession and the War" (editorial), CMA *Journal* 7 (1917): 1011.

44 Macphail diary, 12 May 1916, 65–6.

45 Ibid., 27 Oct. 1915, *et passim* for comments on Jones. On attitudes, see Keirstead, "Doctors at War," 27–38.

46 Morton and Wright, *Second Battle,* 25–30, on medical growth of MHC. Other criticisms are reflected in H.A. Bruce, *Report on the CAMS.* On Thompson, see Morton and Wright, 85.

47 See ibid.; and Desmond Morton: *A Peculiar Kind of Politics: Canada's Overseas Ministry in the First World War* (Toronto: University of Toronto Press 1982), 86–7. See also Hughes to Sir Robert Borden, 2 Sept. 1916, NAC, Borden Papers, OC 311, 33863–5; Perley to Borden, 8 Nov. 1915 on Bruce and secrecy; H.A. Bruce, *Varied Operations* (Toronto: Longmans Green 1958), 86–90.

48 See Bruce, *Report on CAM Service;* Hughes at the Empire Club, Toronto, 9 Nov. 1916 (Toronto *Mail & Empire,* 10 Dec. 1916); Canada House of Commons, *Debates,* 6 Feb. 1917, 538ff.

49 See, for example, Bruce "Surgical Efficiency in an Army Medical Service," CMA *Journal* 9 (1919): 990–2.

50 Reaction and criticism of Bruce's report is found in Macphail, *Medical Services,* 158–72, 180–4; Morton, *Peculiar Politics,* 94–5, 104.

51 Ibid., 105; Macphail, *Medical Services,* 184. On Foster, see Tony Foster, *Meeting of Generals* (Toronto 1986), 1–26.

52 Bruce's view is argued in *Politics and the Canadian Army Medical Corps: A History of Intrigue Containing Many Facts Omitted from the Official Records Showing How Efforts at Rehabilitation Were Balked* (Toronto 1919). On the Smart charges, see Morton, *Peculiar Politics,* 192–4. On continuing controversy, see *Saturday Night,* 29 Mar. 1919; Maj. Gen. G.L. Foster to Sir Edward Kemp, 1 May 1919, NAC, Kemp Papers, file 6a.

53 Solutions of the recruiting problem are discussed in Keirstead, "Doctors at War," 25–7; *Army Medical Corps Instructions no. 165,* 3 Oct. 1916.

54 On Marlow's report, *Special Committee, 1917,* 58–9, 166–80, 182–230; *Canadian Annual Review 1916,* 381 and 1917, 533; "The Marlow Medical Report," MA *Journal* 7 (1917): 252–4; Morton and Wright, *Second Battle,* 85–6; on transfer to CAMC, ibid., 87, 89–90; "Military Hospitals Commission," Adami Papers, NAC RG 9, III B 2, file 3753.

55 Macphail, *Medical Services*, 322; Major C.V. Currie, "History of the CAMC in MD 2," Adami Papers, file 3754; *Canadian Annual Review, 1918*, 560.

56 Cited in Carman, *Return of the Troops*, 99. On the *Llandovery Castle*, see Colonel G.W.L. Nicholson, *Seventy Years of Service: A History of the Royal Canadian Army Medical Corps* (Ottawa: Borealis Press 1977), 105–7; Macphail, *Medical Services*, 241–4.

57 Colonel A. Primrose, "Presidential Address to the Toronto Academy of Medicine," *CMA Journal* 9 (1919): 8–9. Similar views were expressed by the DSCR's Director of Medical Services. See Lt Col. F. McKelvey Bell, "Medical Services of the Department of Soldiers' Civil Re-establishment," ibid., 34–5. See also Morton and Wright, *Second Battle*, 32–6, 57–8, 116.

58 On the policy, see Ernest Scammell, "Canadian Practice in Dealing with Crippled Soldiers," *American Journal of Care for Cripples* 5 (1918); Paul U. Kellogg, "The Battle-Ground for Wounded Men," ibid., 4: 139–67; Major, CAMC (J.L. Todd), "Returned Soldiers and the Medical Profession," *CMA Journal* 7 (1917): 250ff.; Ernest Scammell, *The Provision of Employment for Members of the Canadian Expeditionary Force on Their Return to Canada and the Re-education of Those Who Are Unable To Follow Their Previous Occupation Because of Disability* (Ottawa 1916).

59 For a summary of rehabilitation policies, see Desmond Morton, "Noblest and Best: Retraining Canada's War Disabled," *Journal of Canadian Studies* 16 (1981): 75–85. On Christian, Jaffray, and other notable cases: G.C. Millar, "The Men Who Came Back," *Maclean's*, 1 Dec. 1921.

60 See Morton and Wright, *Second Battle*, 237, for the situation in 1926; Morton, "Resisting the Pension Evil," 205.

61 Ibid., 212–13; Morton and Wright, *Second Battle*, 141–2, 152–3.

62 E. Frances Upton to father, 16 Feb. 1919, Upton Papers (in possession of author). On nurses' problems, see Jean Gunn, "The Service of Canadian Nurses and Voluntary Aides during the War," *Canadian Nurse and Hospital Review* 15 (1919): 1975–6.

63 Colonel E.J. Williams, "The Return of the Army Medical Officers," *CMA Journal* 9 (1919): 221. On the problem and personal choices, Keirstead, "Doctors at War," 242–62. On Banting, see Michael Bliss, *Banting: A Biography* (Toronto: McClelland and Stewart 1984), 48–50. On problems of older doctors, see testimony of Dr Maxwell Inglis, Canada House of Commons, *Proceedings of the Special Committee on Pensions* 1920, 192–6; Maj. Gen. J.T. Fotheringham to Major Harley Smith, 23 Sept. 1919, Fotheringham Papers, file 16.

64 Colonel J.L. Biggar, "State Medicine and Rehabilitation," *CMA Journal* 9 (1918): 1015.

65 Todd, "Meaning of Rehabilitation," 5. See also editorial, CMA *Journal* 9 (1919): 175, 275; P.H. Bryce, "The Medical and Allied Professions as a State Service," ibid., 9 (1921): 71ff. For an overview, see Naylor, *Private Practice, Public Payment*, 26–57. For a sympathetic American view, see W.J. Monaghan in *American Medicine* 25 (1919): 316 *et passim*.

66 Naylor, *Private Practice, Public Payment*, 58–66. The subject is reviewed by Robert S. Bothwell and John R. English, "Pragmatic Physicians: Canadian Medicine and Health-Care Insurance, 1919–1945," in Shortt, *Medicine in Canadian Society*. See also Naylor, *Private Practice, Public Payment*, 58–66.

67 *Toronto Daily Star*, 3 Mar. 1919.

68 Adami, "Medicine and the War," 882.

69 Dr Glen T. Hamilton, abstract of the presidential Address at the Annual Meeting of the Manitoba Medical Association, CMA *Journal* 13 (1923): 151.

70 For example, see C.L. Starr, "Laurence Bruce Robertson B.A., M.D.," ibid., 13 (1923): 216, on the application of transfusion to the care of severely burned infants. See also George E. Armstrong, "The Influence of the War on Surgery, Civil or Military," ibid., 9 (1919): 396–405; *Toronto Daily Star*, 1–2 Mar. 1919.

71 Bernard Langdon Wyatt, "Industrial Medicine," CMA *Journal* 13 (1923): 114. See also Wyatt, "Industrial Medicine: Its Motives and Merits," CMA *Journal* 13 (1923): 662 *et passim*; Keirstead, "Doctors at War," 268–70.

72 Ibid., 273–7.

The Development of Neuropsychiatry in the Canadian Army (Overseas) 1939–1943

TERRY COPP

The impact of the Second World War upon the Canadian medical profession has not been seriously investigated. Yet for thousands of Canadian doctors and nurses the war was to be a major formative influence in their professional lives. Service in the armed forces brought medical professionals under direct state authority, and the military discipline imposed upon them required adaptation to life in a complex bureaucratic system that was quite unlike any other organization they had previously encountered. Adaptation was also required by the agency of the state that employed them, the Department of National Defence. This examination of the origin and growth of neuropsychiatry in the Canadian army is offered as a case-study of the relationship between the medical profession and the army. It suggests that at least in the case of neuropsychiatry the medical profession was equal to the task of imposing its own priorities and values on the state.

The Royal Canadian Army Medical Corps, like all other branches of the Canadian Armed Services, was magnificently unprepared for the Second World War. As late as November 1939 there were only forty-two medical officers and eleven nursing sisters in the permanent army.[1] But unlike other branches of the armed services, which would have to train most of their recruits in the elementary arts of war, the RCAMC could draw upon its militia units and indeed upon the medical community at large with the certain knowledge that its key volunteers would already be professionally trained.

The problem was to organize that expertise in a manner that would advance the war effort. Initially there was little evidence that the medical corps was capable of doing this. The system of medical examination for recruits had changed little since the First World War, and despite representations from the medical community, no provisions were made for routine chest X-rays, urinalysis, or Wassermann tests. It was also decided that it would not be necessary to employ specialists on medical boards because, "in any instance where a specialist's report is considered necessary to establish a candidate's fitness, the individual should be rejected by the board."[2]

Criticism of the army's methods of examining volunteers came from all directions, and before the end of 1939 re-examination of all recruits was ordered. Now there would be a chest X-ray, chemical urinalysis, and a more detailed physical.[3] The question of psychological testing for the selection and classification of army personnel was also considered. A conference on "The Use of Psychological Methods in Wartime," held in Ottawa on 2 October 1939, concluded that "it would be advisable to introduce into the recruiting examinations, intelligence and aptitude tests"[4] and urged that the director general of Medical Services (DGMS) be asked to co-operate with the Canadian Psychological Association, which had offered to devise and implement the tests.

The chairman of the conference was Canada's most distinguished scientist, Sir Frederick Banting, and prominent among the advocates of testing at the meeting was Major General A.L.G. McNaughton, president of the National Research Council. McNaughton had been chief of General Staff from 1929 until 1935, and in early October he was anxiously awaiting the call to return to the colours. When the call came, however, it was to take up the post of "Inspector-General of the units of 1st Canadian Division" with a view to commanding the Red Patch Division when it was sent overseas, not to the senior administrative position in the army.

Without McNaughton's direct involvement, psychological testing stook little chance of making headway in the army. The chief of the General Staff, Major-General T.V. Anderson, and the adjutant-general, Major General H.H. Matthews, showed no interest in the idea. Neither the senior medical officer, Colonel J.L. Potter, nor his successor as DGMS, Brigadier B.M. Gorrsline, would voluntarily have anything to do with "psychological methods." Indeed, a meeting of psychiatrists called to discuss approaches to psychiatric problems in the army was flatly told that "there would be no testing and no psychiatric screen at enlistment."[5] The examining boards were to "reject obvious misfits, subsequently unit medical officers were to make their diagnosis and refer difficult cases to regional consultants for disposal."[6] When new instructions to medical boards were issued in early 1940, doctors were told to establish "that the recruit is sufficiently intelligent" by questioning him. Obvious misfits were defined as those "with a history of nervous breakdown ... residence in an institution ... drug addiction ... or a family history indicating nervous instability such as migraine, eccentricity etc."[7]

The general lack of concern for intelligence testing, not to mention any form of personality evaluation, fairly reflected the attitude towards psychology and psychiatry in the Canadian medical profession. The overwhelming majority of doctors inside or outside the army sincerely believed that any well-trained physician could evaluate an individual's ability or stability as well as any psychiatrist and better than any psychologist. Psychologists were not even medical doctors! If the medical board had doubts about an individual's mental fitness, its job was to reject, not to diagnose him.

There is a good case to be made for this point of view, but it is evident that during the early fall of 1939, when more than fifty thousand Canadians enlisted in the army, the overworked medical boards did not take the time to evaluate seriously all of the volunteers. A number of individuals with a history of mental illness,[8] as well as a much larger group of mentally deficient recruits, were enrolled in the army as category A or B personnel, the two classifications that placed no limitations on military service.

The attitude of the RCAMC towards intelligence testing and psychiatric screening was clear enough, but what did the corps intend to do with psychiatric casualties produced by the stress of war? The Canadian army had admitted to 15,500 "neuropsychiatric disabilities" in the First World War – 9,000 of them diagnosed as "shell shock and neurosis";[9] it had to be assumed that similar casualties would occur again. In fact, the RCAMC had not developed any scheme. But the director-general of Medical Services and ultimately the minister of Defence acted quickly enough when Dr Colin Russel approached the army with a plan for establishing a neurosurgical, neurological, and neuropsychiatric hospital that would go to France as a specialized unit in the Canadian expeditionary force.

The contrast between the army's resistance to psychological testing and its affirmative response to Dr Russel was a measure of the status Russel possessed in the Canadian medical profession. A graduate of McGill (MD 1901), Russel had been encouraged to study neurology and psychiatry at Johns Hopkins, then under the direction of William Osler. After leaving Baltimore he spent several years in Zurich, Berlin, and Paris, working with the leading continental neurologists. In 1905 he interned at the National Hospital for the Relief and Cure of the Paralysed and Epileptic. The National Hospital, or simply "Queen Square," after its location in London, was the mecca of twentieth-century neurology, and when Russel returned to Montreal he was able to establish himself as a leading figure in what was, for Canada, a relatively new clinical specialization.

Russel had volunteered for the medical corps in the First World War, and by 1917 he was in charge of neuropsychiatry at Granville Special Hospital for Nervous Cases, a Canadian army establishment at Ramsgate in England. Russel published a number of articles on his experiences with "shell-shock" patients and was regarded as something of an expert on the subject. After the war he became clinical professor of neurology at McGill, and in 1934 he joined Wilder Penfield as chief neurologist at the Montreal Neurological Institute.[11] In the late thirties Penfield's MNI was a world-famous centre of neurosurgery, and Russel's reputation was further enhanced by his association with Penfield. In fact Penfield was no particular admirer of Russel's and was deeply disappointed when Colin Russel, rather than Wilder Penfield, was authorized to organize a specialized unit for overseas service.[12]

Russel was brought back into the army as a lieutenant-colonel with the title of "consultant neuropsychiatrist." He had very definite views on the origin and proper treatment of neuroses, views that he outlined in a paper published in the *Canadian Medical Association Journal* for December 1939. Despite the fact that Russel had never been near the front lines, he was confident that all fear reactions – "anxiety, trembling and jumpiness ... mental confusion or even almost a stupour" – could be handled with "common sense treatment of rest, food and an understanding appreciation."[13] Such men, he believed, could be returned to duty in a few days. The real problem, and the task of the neuropsychiatrist, was the treatment of "a large class, which became larger, the further one got away from the front [who] exhibited all the evidences of conversion hysteria – the so-called shell shock." Russel also knew how to deal with these cases. Hysteria is the "great simulator," he wrote, and it can involve "blindness in one or both eyes, mutism, associated or not with deafness, convulsions of a major or minor type ... profuse sweating ... paralyzed extremities ... or a host of other manifestations ... I have seen examples of all of these and cleared them up by purely psychic treatment, and very quickly."[14]

The cause of such hysteria was either an "extraordinary suggestibility" or the absence of "high moral standards." It could be cured by the use of faradism (that is, the application of an electric current until the patient abandoned his hysteria), isolation, or – and this was a special feature of Russel's treatment program in the Second

World War – the use of the "wire brush."[15] (The wire brush, charged with an asymmetric alternating current, was applied to the "paralyzed" limb.) With these methods, Russel claimed, "I was able to return over 71.4 per cent back to full duty ... The cure of a psychoneuropath really consists of a mental contest resulting in the victory of the physician. This, in conclusion, is the secret of psychotherapy."[16]

Russel also wanted the hospital staff to include two neurosurgical teams, both of which would be mobile, using specially fitted vehicles that "Mr. McLaughlin of Oshawa"[17] was preparing. The connection between Russel's special hospital for the treatment of war neuroses, to be located "in the zone of the army where strict discipline is maintained,"[18] and a neurosurgical unit may not seem overwhelmingly obvious, but the link was clear to him. The army's neurological hospital was to be modelled on the MNI, where neurologists and neurosurgeons were grouped together in an institution separate from general surgery or medicine. In the pre-war world of Canadian academic medicine the treatment of neuroses in hospitals was the exclusive province of neurologists, who, if they were interested in neuroses, described themselves as neuropsychiatrists. If the neurologists were to be grouped with the neurosurgeons, then the neurological hospital would of necessity be the non-custodial psychiatric hospital.

This approach was unique to McGill, where Wilder Penfield had created his institute with Rockefeller money. At the Toronto General, neurosurgery was very much part of general surgery, just as neurology (and neuropsychiatry) were firmly wedded to general medicine. Dr Kenneth McKenzie, who, like Penfield, had worked with the great neurosurgical pioneer Harvey Cushing, had begun his neurosurgical service at Toronto General in 1924. By 1939 he and his colleagues at Toronto were convinced that their approach to neurosurgery and neurology was the correct one.[19] McKenzie did not believe it made any sense to divide up surgical specializations, especially in wartime, when multiple wounds could be expected. What, he asked, "would be the procedure in cases where wounds of the abdomen or chest were associated with wounds of the spinal cord and consequent paralysis?"[20] McKenzie's arguments were not only difficult to answer; his approach to neurosurgery fitted in with the British army plan. Ultimately, his model prevailed in the war zone, with neurosurgery and neuropsychiatry units attached to base hospitals. A small mobile "group," No. 1 Mobile Neurosurgical Unit, was introduced into the field in late 1944 under the command of one of McKenzie's colleagues, Bill Keith. It was similar in function to the "Head Unit" established in the British army by Hugh Cairns, not to Russel's 1939 proposal.

All this was in the future. In 1939 Russel met McKenzie's criticisms with the prestige of Wilder Penfield. At a meeting chaired by Brigadier Gorrsline, Penfield, his close associate William Cone, and Colin Russel answered Mckenzie's questions with the statement that general surgeons could be brought to the neurological hospital. Their scheme, Penfield insisted, allowed for "the cooperation and teamwork of neurologists and neurosurgeons which, in the Montreal Neurological Institute, we find of such mutual advantage."[21] The meeting concluded with "agreement" that the special unit, to be called "No. 1 Neurological and Neurosurgical Hospital," would take the field with the Canadian troops scheduled for France.

The Montrealers had prevailed, but the hospital could not function without the assistance of Toronto doctors. William Cone was to be senior neurosurgeon, with Harry Botterell from Toronto as his "second." Russel was the senior neuropsychiatrist, with H.H. Hyland from Toronto General Hospital next in rank. The junior neurologists were Fred Hanson, a young American who was working at the MNI when war broke out,[22] and Clifford Richardson, a Toronto neurologist who combined experience as a house physician at Queen Square with work at the Tavistock Clinic and the London Institute of Psychoanalysis. In 1939 neither man knew very much about "shell shock" or the military; enlistment, in Richardson's words, "was just the natural thing to do." Richardson, who had gone on a walking tour of Germany in 1936 and been amazed by the atmosphere of Hitler's Reich, was clear on the "threat and danger of Nazi philosophy" and was certain that such "a fanatic leader, such dangerous ideas had to be stopped."[23]

For Richardson and the other volunteers the winter of 1939–40 offered the opportunity to practise that supreme military virtue – patience. The First Division with its medical units arrived in England just before Christmas. Quartered at Aldershot in ancient barrack buildings without central heating, the whole force seemed to catch influenza or colds. An outbreak of German measles compounded the misery, and Colonel R.M. Luton, the senior medical officer overseas, made arrangements for Canadian soldiers to be admitted to British army hospitals.[24] When the medical staff for the first two Canadian general hospitals arrived in February 1940, there were no buildings for them to work in and there was no particular need for their services. Discussions between Ottawa and London centred on the medical establishment required for the Canadian units going to France to join the British Expeditionary Force. National Defence headquarters seemed quite incapable of coming to a clear decision on this question, but it was agreed that the group of neurologists and neurosurgeons who were beginning to be called "No. 1 Nuts" were intended for the war zone in France and could, therefore, be sent overseas.[25]

Colin Russel, Bill Cone, and Harry Botterell left for London in May 1940 and arrived just as the evacuation from Dunkirk was taking place.[26] The First Canadian Division would not be going to France in the foreseeable future, and the priority attached to sending the Neurological Hospital overseas had presumably ended. Cone and Botterell kept busy with research at Queen Square while Russel worked to keep his hospital idea alive. Lord Camrose, the proprietor of the *Daily Telegraph*, offered his country home, Hackwood Park, a spacious mansion near Basingstoke in Hampshire, to Russel, and somehow he persuaded the army authorities in London to authorize the agreement. No one in Canada had thought to cancel the move of the rest of the hospital staff, and in September of 1940 No. 1 Neurological Hospital, usually simply called Basingstoke, opened for business as a two-hundred-bed hospital. The nurses, twelve from the MNI and eight from Toronto, under Matron Myra Mac-Donald,[27] were housed in the Camrose family rooms while the doctors settled into the servants' quarters. Construction of Nissen huts for additional wards began, and the hospital community settled into a routine.

The minister of National Defence, J.L. Ralston, eventually noticed the hospital's existence when the costs of establishing the unit were brought to his attention. Why, he asked, was a unit designed for service in France developing into a new and expensive stationary hospital in England?[28] Colonel Luton's reply argued that "the hospital will accompany our expeditionary force to the field when the time comes" and "it would be an error to dissolve a unit upon which a great deal of money ($50,000) had been expended."[29] The idea of sending the hospital overseas was not formally abandoned until 1942, when it was agreed that new methods of evacuation and treatment made the original role of the hospital "undesirable."[30] By that time Basingstoke had acquired a vital role as both an army hospital and an emergency medical services hospital for the county of Hampshire. No. 1 Neurological was in place for the duration.

Basingstoke was well placed to receive patients from Southhampton and other English port cities devastated by the Blitz of 1940–41. In addition the neurosurgeons found steady work because the army had seen fit to give large numbers of young Canadians the opportunity to ride high-powered motorcycles on the "wrong side" of

narrow roads even under black-out conditions. The resulting may-
hem was such that German propaganda broadcasts demanded a
motorcycle for every Canadian soldier.[31]

Motorcycle accidents also produced a number of post-traumatic
syndromes that required the staff to exercise all their skill in determining whether a physical basis for the condition existed. Epilepsy
was, however, "the most common 'organic' condition encountered"
and required careful investigation. A diagnosis of epilepsy was automatic grounds for return to Canada, and many epileptics had tried
to conceal their condition by taking anti-convulsants or relying on
the protection of friends. Neurosyphilis, sciatica, neuritis, migraine,
and narcolepsy were also encountered, but it was obvious from the
first weeks that the main work of No. 1 Nuts would be with patients
requiring the attention of the neuropsychiatrists.[32]

Diagnosis and treatment of neuropsychiatric cases was under the
direction of Colin Russel until repeated bouts of illness, which he
attributed to his age and the English winter, led him to request a
return to Canada in early 1942.[33] Russel was most interested in the
cases of conversion hysteria, which closely resembled the kind of
shell shock he had dealt with in the First World War. The old treatment with the electric wire brush was used by Russel with a few of
these patients,[34] but simple psychotherapy, reclassification, or reas-
signment, was usually all that was required. Most of the patients
admitted to Basingstoke were suffering from psychoneuroses manifested in a wide variety of symptoms – strong fear reactions, chronic
headaches, enuresis, gastric illness, uncontrollable restlessness, ex-
aggerated physical weakness, muscle tics, obsessions, phobias – the
list is almost endless.

H.H. Hyland, who had considerable experience with similar patients at Toronto General Hospital, established the basic routines in
psychiatric treatment. Hyland had joined Dr Goldwin Howland's
neurological service at Toronto General Hospital in 1930. Ward G,
with 20 to 30 beds for organic neurological disease and 25 to 40 beds
for nervous and mental disease, was the largest neurological and
psychiatric service in Canada and the model for most of the country.[35] Hyland had been trained in neurology at Queen Square, but
he had developed a strong interest in psychiatry. He approached
the problem of mental illness with the neurologist's conviction that
there was a "physiological basis of mental functions and dysfunc-
tions,"[36] but he maintained that "any personality disorder is comprised of the given personality (and the physical substratum) as
inherited and moulded by environmental influences reacting to a
certain group of circumstances which arise at a given time." The

differences between "normal," "neurotic," and "psychotic" disorders were, he wrote, "narrow and ill-defined." The symptoms of mental stress "also occur in varying degrees in normal persons. In others these same symptoms tend to be carried to such an extreme as to merit the term neurotic."

Hyland's undogmatic, practical approach to psychiatry was generally shared by his junior colleagues, although Richardson and Hanson were much less committed to the virtues of psychotherapy. Richardson had become thoroughly disenchanted with psychoanalytically influenced psychiatry while working at the Tavistock Clinic and attending sessions at the London Institute of Psychoanalysis in the mid-thirties. He had little confidence that anything could be done with the hundreds of patients who arrived at Basingstoke with long records of neurotic reactions to the stress of civilian and army life and was quite certain that "return to Canada and discharge" was the correct procedure for chronic neurotics as well as psychopaths and alcoholics.[37] This view sometimes led to difficulties. On one occasion, "Ric," as Richardson was always called, told a chronic bed-wetter that he would be "returned to Canada." By next morning word had spread and the holding unit stank of urine.[38]

The number of "reboardings" in the Canadian army was causing the military authorities some concern by 1941. In the period February 1940 to March 1941, 2,135 troops of all ranks were returned to Canada as Category E, and 21 per cent of these were classified as mental cases, "chiefly anxiety neuroses, chronic alcoholism or mental deficiency."[39] In addition to these 453 individuals returned to Canada, hundreds of other Canadian soldiers were or had been neuropsychiatric patients at No. 1 Neurological Hospital and No. 15 General Hospital. The problem began to reach epidemic proportions in the winter of 1941, and Colonel R.M. Luton, the senior medical officer overseas, appointed a Committee on Cases of Anxiety Neurosis[40] to try to develop policy.

The committee met at Basingstoke on 13 January 1941. The first order of business was to change the name of the committee and the scope of its investigation. Since the whole range of mental illness was to be examined, the title "Functional Nervous Diseases" was adopted and the "Official Nomenclature of Diseases 1931" used to enumerate the five diagnostic categories: mental deficiency; chronic alcoholism and drug addition; functional psychoses; psychopathic personalities; and psychoneuroses.

The committee decided that the "higher grade of defectives ... would be able to perform routine tasks quite efficiently"[41] and should only be discharged if they had behaviour problems that did not respond to army discipline. Drug addicts, chronic alcoholics, and functional psychotics were to be returned to Canada forthwith.

The broad category of psychopathic personalities was also easily disposed of.[42] Generally neuropsychiatrists used this term to encompass a variety of chronic "social misfits" who had been arrested for burglary, larceny, petty theft, robbery with violence, homosexuality, and absence without leave. These individuals came to Basingstoke on referral from various prisons and detention barracks. They were to be returned to Canada and discharged from the service unless there was clear evidence that they would respond to military discipline.

This left the largest category, the psychoneuroses, to be dealt with. Major Hyland, as the senior neuropsychiatrist (Colin Russel was absent due to illness), presented the case for the retention and treatment of all anxiety and hysteria cases. At Basingstoke a good deal of attention was paid to each patient,[43] with treatment "initiated by a careful evaluation of physical, psychological and sociological components." A detailed case-history, with "questioning about childhood environmental influences, parental attitudes and relationships, phobias, school and work record, disposition towards sports and physical dangers, sexual habits, adaptation to difficulties, mood changes, details of army experiences etc.," followed a thorough physical. A systematic mental examination "surveying intellect as well as emotion" was carried out, and a detailed discussion of the factors "causing the immediate mental conflict and tension" was undertaken with each patient. Hyland believed in repeated talks with patients so that "repressed fears and conflicts" could be aired again and again. The immediate problems that had caused or at least precipitated the neurosis were to be dealt with where possible, but when the problem was insoluble Hyland urged a "philosophical outlook" and the avoidance of continued "emotional thinking." In selected cases "hypnosis, sodium pentathol suggestion by use of faradism and occasionally prolonged narcosis" were used.

Hyland's argument for intensive treatment of all psychoneurotics was challenged by Major F.H. Van Nostrand, the neuropsychiatrist from the Canadian army's No. 15 General Hospital at Bramshott. Van Nostrand expressed the view that "the majority of these soldiers were of little use, even when they returned to their unit." In this opinion, slight strain would probably cause them to break down again. Hyland replied that individuals who "responded to psychotherapy should be given another opportunity to carry on with their unit." If they broke down a second time, "they could be brought before a medical board for reclassification."[45] The committee agreed to postpone a policy decision until follow-up studies of patients returned to their units from both hospitals could be undertaken.

F.H. Van Nostrand had come to RCAMC from a very different background from Hyland's. Van Nostrand had served in the First World War as a stretcher-bearer and then joined the Royal Flying Corps. Between the wars he had devoted his energies to rebuilding the family farm north of Toronto while acquiring a medical degree. Van Nostrand joined the staff of Christie Street Hospital for Veterans when he graduated, and for the next ten years he dealt with a wide variety of psychoneurotic patients.[46] For "Van" psychotherapy was applied common sense; you tried to get the individual to face up to his problems and function as best he could.[47] The majority of patients at Bramshott, like those at Basingstoke, had long histories of pre-war problems, and many had been in and out of mental institutions.[48] Van Nostrand was quite certain that intensive psychotherapy would have little lasting impact on such men. He also believed that a second group of soldiers, who had developed neurotic symptoms in England without exposure to combat, were failing to cope with the normal stress of army life. If they could not be dealt with effectively by regimental medical officers, chaplains, or their unit COs, it was unlikely that hospitalization and diagnosis as neurotics would accomplish anything. Indeed, it was probable that such treatment would reinforce a patient's sense of himself as a person who was sick.[49]

The follow-up studies took a very long time to complete. But a preliminary report based on sixty-five case-histories of men who had no previous history of mental instability was made available by Hyland in October of 1941. The Committee on Functional Nervous Diseases was told "that out of 65 cases which had been returned to their units for an average of three months, 70.2% of the in-patients and 43.7% of the out-patients were doing full duty efficiently and without complaint." Hyland also told the committee that he had studied fifty-four other patients who had not been returned to duty and he was struck by "the frequency of a poor family and personal history as a background in these cases." The committee, after some discussion, decided that those cases that showed a "bad personal and family history" should be recategorized and sent home, while those "who have a good background and respond well to treatment"[51] should be returned to duty.

A more detailed study of patients from Basingstoke was produced by Richardson in April 1942. During an eighteen-month period the hospital had admitted 1,171 psychiatric cases, of which 649 were diagnosed as psychoneurosis. Of these, 55 per cent were returned to duty. The follow-up study was able to obtain "adequate information" on only 75 of these men. The data on this group gave a different impression from that conveyed by the earlier report, for just 25 per cent of the men "remained well and efficient during periods of three to fifteen months after discharge to duty."[52] If the 75 cases were in any way representative, the Canadian army was not decreasing "wastage" very effectively. Richardson was disturbed by these statistics, but he attributed the high failure rate to the large number of patients who "should never have been taken into the army because of nervous instability"[53] and pointed out that British army experience with psychoneurosis was very similar.

British experience with mental disorders among soldiers who had not been exposed to combat was indeed strikingly similar. More than one hundred thousand men had been medically boarded out of the army in the first year of the war with gastric, mental, and nervous problems,[54] and thousands more had been treated and returned to duty with an uncertain prognosis. The extent of the problem had led to an acrimonious public debate that took place in *The Lancet* and other leading medical journals. Calls for an end to civilian doctors treating soldiers were made on the grounds that "the Englishmen regards soldiering as terribly hard for the poor boys: and at the slightest opportunity pampering the soldier becomes a favourite pastime."[55]

Complaints about malingering and "skrimshanking" were also common, but the central focus of the professional debate was between those who doubted that the "neurotic could be freed of his neurotic tendencies"[56] and those who were confident that psychotherapy could return a significant proportion of soldiers to full duty. *The Lancet* came down strongly on the side of those who favoured rigidly excluding all neurotics from the armed forces. An editorial of September 1940 flatly declared that, with a rigorous policy, the army "would no doubt lose some valuable soldiers, but it would be rid of some thousands of men who are of no use to it at all."[57] The British army, struggling to obtain its share of manpower in an unequal competition with the air force and navy,[58] was unwilling to adopt this attitude. The consulting psychiatrist to British Army at Home, Brigadier John R. Rees, had come into the Royal Army Medical Corps from his position as medical director of the Tavistock Clinic, an institute of human relations committed to social psychiatry in the broadest sense. Rees and the psychiatrists he brought into the service with him were strongly committed to a treatment approach that emphasized various types of therapies – psychological and occupational. Ultimately the British army even established a separate facility for the intensive retraining of psychoneurotics.[59]

The Canadian neuropsychiatrists at Basingstoke were divided on the question. Van Nostrand was firmly on the side of *The Lancet*, as was Richardson, but Hyland remained committed to a treatment model. Psychiatric views were, however, irrelevant. The Canadian army was simply not willing to accept the notion that large numbers of men should be returned to Canada when all signs pointed to a looming manpower shortage. No. 1 Neurological Hospital would continue to function as a treatment centre for the more severe neurotic cases and a custodial centre for psychotics awaiting shipment back to Canada. A strong effort was made to encourage regimental medical officers to keep mild psychoneurotic cases with their units; if referral to a psychiatrist was necessary, then they were to be seen at Basingstoke on an out-patient basis before admission was considered. The work of treating psychoneuroses at the hospital continued throughout the war but with little sign of any breakthrough in recovery rates.

The time, energy, and scarce resources devoted to the treatment of neuroses in the Canadian army may seem disproportionate in view of the poor results, but there are other considerations. The army's concern for reducing wastage provided an environment in which the medical personnel were encouraged to devote considerable attention to soldiers as individuals. Quite apart from the moral value of this approach, there is some evidence that it was important in a more direct way. Among the men returned to duty in 1941 was a young officer[60] who spent four weeks at Basingstoke under treatment for anxiety neurosis with conversion symptoms. Released to his unit, he had to return to the hospital after a short stint of regimental duty. The second treatment session was much shorter, and this time the young man was able to stick it out, acquiring self-confidence and developing into one of the handful of outstanding senior combatant officers in the Canadian army. It might well be argued that No. 1 Neurological justified its existence on this case alone.

During 1942 the hospital at Basingstoke continued to expand, with huts occupying more and more space on the vast lawns of Hackwood Park. Van Nostrand was transferred to No. 1 Neurological as the new commanding officer, and in June Colin Russel, now almost sixty-five years of age, returned to McGill. Herbert Hyland was the senior neuropsychiatrist overseas, but Canadian military headquarters offered Russel's job as consulting neuropsychiatrist (and the promotion to full colonel) to Van Nostrand. Shortly afterwards Hyland returned to Canada and his work at Toronto General Hospital. Richardson became the senior neuropsychiatrist at Basingstoke. The expansion of psychiatric services into every part of the Canadian army would take place under the direction of Van Nostrand and Richardson, two men of outstanding ability who worked together easily for the remainder of the war.

Two other McGill men left Basingstoke along with Russel in 1942. William Cone returned to Montreal Neurological, and Fred Hanson joined the American army. Hanson had been restless at No. 1 Nuts and had sought out action in some bizarre ways, including taking part in motor-torpedo-boat raids in the Channel.[61] In May 1942 he transferred to the American army at the request of the senior medical officer in the European Theater of Operations. Hanson became the unofficial adviser on neuropsychiatric problems in an army that had not yet recognized their existence. He was able to gain permission to join the Second Canadian Division for the Dieppe raid "to observe the stress of actual combat," and then actively sought a role in the North African campaign. He reached the front in Tunisia during March 1943 and was able to initiate the development of front-line treatment for combat neuropsychiatric casualties. Hanson's brilliant record in organizing psychiatric facilities in Tunisia and developing immediate treatment procedures led to his appointment as consultant in Neuropsychiatry, North African Theater. Later in 1943 he played a major role in establishing a complete system of psychiatric services for the American army,[62] a system based on the lessons learned at Basingstoke.

The Canadian army's neuropsychiatric tradition, with its emphasis on keeping psychiatry with neurology and general medicine, was a uniquely Canadian development. In the British army psychiatry was linked with personnel selection and psychology rather than the medical services, and RCAMC physicians frequently ignored the advice of the specialist in psychological medicine. The Canadian system was also unique in having a single central institution, the hospital at Basingstoke, to serve as a training centre for all psychiatrists in the overseas army. The short course at Basingstoke, which preceded all appointments to work in the field, provided Canadian doctors with a common approach to psychiatric problems in the army. For many, No. 1 Neurological Hospital provided stimulating post-graduate education of a type that few Depression-era physicians had previously experienced. The neuropsychiatric hospital was much admired by British and American medical men because medical rather than military priorities seemed to predominate in the Canadian army.

This was an accurate reading until the middle of 1942, but pressures from Canadian Military Headquarters in England redirected army psychiatry towards personnel selection, and for a time resources were shifted away from Basingstoke. Richardson protested this change in priorities, arguing that the "chronic shortage of medical officers"[63] at the hospital was severely handicapping the treatment program. His complaints and the steady increase in the supply of new "baby psychiatrists"[64] made it possible to reverse the trend during the latter half of 1943. The arrival of Dr Allan Walters at Basingstoke symbolized this renewal. Walters, a neuropsychiatrist from Toronto General, was a man of enormous energy. He was thoroughly trained in neurology, but his real interest was in psychiatry. An enthusiastic pioneer in physical treatment methods, especially insulin sub-coma therapy, he also embraced Freudian-influenced psychotherapy.[65] Walters took over direction of the neurosis wards at Basingstoke, and in the last two years of the war dozens of Canadian doctors were introduced to psychiatry through the short course at Basingstoke. A small group of energetic physicians had created a unique Canadian institution in the heart of England. It was one of the most successful marriages of the medical profession with the state in Canadian history, and a crucial episode in the development of the profession of psychiatry in Canada.

NOTES

The author wishes to acknowledge the support provided by a Hannah Institute grant-in-aid of research.

1 W.R. Feasby, *Official History of the Canadian Medical Services 1939–1945*, vol. 1, *Organization and Campaigns* (Ottawa 1956), 8.
2 Ibid., 34.
3 Ibid., 51.
4 W.R. Feasby, *Official History*, vol. 2, *Clinical Subjects* (Ottawa 1953), 100.
5 Interview, Jack Griffin, Toronto, 25 Oct. 1982.
6 Feasby, 2:56.
7 *General Instructions for the Medical Examination of Recruits for the CASF and NPAM* (Ottawa: King's Printer 1940).
8 National Archives of Canada (NAC) RG 24, vol. 12620.
9 J.P.S. Cathcart, "The Neuro Psychiatric Branch of the Department Civil Re-Establishment," *Ontario Journal of Neuro-Psychiatry* 8 (1928): 46.
10 Details from F.L. McNaughton, "Colin Russel, A Pioneer of Canadian Neurology," *Canadian Medical Association Journal* 77 (1957): 719–23.

11 Jefferson Lewis, *Something Hidden: A Biography of Wilder Penfield* (Toronto: Doubleday 1981), 114–17.

12 Ibid., 163.

13 Colin K. Russel, "The Nature of War Neuroses," CMAJ 41 (1939): 550.

14 Ibid., 533.

15 C. Russel, "A Study of Certain Psychogenetic Conditions among Soldiers," CMAJ 7 (1917): 711.

16 Russel, "The Nature of War Neuroses," 544.

17 Memorandum, Russel to DGMS, 8 Dec. 1939, Russel Papers, Osler Library, McGill University, vol. 3.

18 Memorandum, Lt Col. Colin Russel to DGMS, 31 Oct. 1939, Russel Papers, vol. 3.

19 E. Harry Botterell, "Kenneth George McKenzie, MD, FRCS 1923–1963," *Surgical Neurology* 17, no. 2, (1982): 82–9; and Botterell interview, 30 Oct. 1986.

20 Memorandum, Russel to DGMS, 8 Dec. 1939.

21 Ibid. The meeting ended with "Drs. Penfield and Cone both expressing themselves strongly in favour of the Combined Neurological and Neurosurgical Unit."

22 See A.J. Glass, ed., *Neuropsychiatry in World War II*, vol. 2, *Overseas Theatres* (Washington: Office of the Surgeon General 1973), chap. 1.

23 Richardson interview.

24 Feasby, 1:98.

25 Ibid., 99.

26 Botterell interview.

27 Memorandum, Russel, n.d., Russel Papers.

28 Ralston Papers, vol. 54, file "No. 1 Neurological Hospital, Jan. 1941."

29 R.M. Luton to Senior Officer, CMHQ, 21 Dec. 1940, NAC RG 24, vol. 12583.

30 F.H. Van Nostrand to Luton, 1 May 1942, NAC RG 24, vol. 12604.

31 There are a number of versions of this story. I have made no attempt to track down the correct one. It is perhaps worth recording that 45 per cent of the neurosurgical cases admitted to Basingstoke were accident victims. H. Elliott, "Head Wounds Canadian Army, World War II," *Treatment Services Bulletin*, Aug. 1949, 10.

32 Feasby, 2:60.

33 Russel to DMS, CMHQ, 11 Jan. 1942, vol. 4, Russel Papers.

34 McNaughton, "Colin Russel," 722.

35 F. Somers, "A History of Psychiatry at the Toronto General Hospital," ts, Griffin-Greenland Archives, Toronto, 31–2.

36 The quotations in this paragraph are from H.H. Hyland and J.C. Richardson, "Psychoneurosis in the Canadian Army Overseas," CMAJ 47 (1942): 432–43.

37 Richardson and Botterell interviews.
38 Botterell interview.
39 J.M. Hitsman, "The Problem of Personnel Selection in the Canadian Army Overseas 1939–1946," Report 64, Historical Section CMHQ, 1946, ts, Directorate of History, Dept of National Defence, 4.
40 Minutes, Committee on Cases of Anxiety Neurosis, CASF, 3 Feb. 1941, Russel papers, vol. 4.
41 Ibid.
42 Ibid.
43 This account of treatment at Basingstoke is based on Hyland and Richardson, "Psychoneurosis," 20–1. All quotes in the paragraph are from this article.
44 Minutes, Committee on Cases of Anxiety Neurosis, 3 Feb. 1941.
45 Ibid.
46 Obituary, Dr. Frederick Harold Van Nostrand, CMAJ 113 (1975): 432, and interview with Dr Peter Van Nostrand. Dr Van Nostrand had been recommended to Russel as a neuropsychiatrist when No. 1 Neurological Unit was formed, but Russel had selected doctors with stronger academic credentials. Dr G.F. Boyer to Russel, 25 Nov. 1939, Russel Papers, vol. 7.
47 Van Nostrand interview. Two of "Van's" oldest friends, Dr Bill Keith and Dr Bill White, were present during this interview. Both tried to explain Van Nostrand's practical, common-sense approach to me.
48 Appendix B, "Report on Selection of Personnel and Mental Disease in the Canadian Army Overseas," 18 July 1941, NAC RG 24, vol. 2, 12620, file 31.
49 Van Nostrand repeatedly expressed these views in reports and memoranda throughout the war.
50 Report of 8 July 1941, 2.
51 Minutes, Committee on Functional Nervous Disease, 31 Oct. 1941, NAC RG 24, vol. 12620.
52 Hyland and Richardson, "Psychoneurosis," 22–3.
53 J.C. Richardson, "Psychoneurosis in the CASF," NAC RG 24, vol. 12620.
54 The Lancet, editorial of 26 Apr. 1941, 530.
55 Ibid., letter of 20 July 1940, 82.
56 G. Debenham, Denis Hill, Will Sargant, Elliot Slater, "Treatment of War Neuroses," in ibid., 25 Jan. 1941, 107.
57 Ibid., editorial of 7 Sept. 1940, 299.
58 J.R. Rees, "Three Years of Military Psychiatry," British Journal of Medicine, 2 Jan. 1943, 4278. Rees writes, "The Royal Navy and Royal Air Force have priority of choice and the Civilian Defence Services have claimed a great many men. The Army comes last in the list ... [and]

... has therefore to deal with very considerable numbers of dull, neurotic and unstable men."

59 Northfield Military Hospital, Birmingham, opened in April 1942 with a 200-bed Hospital Wing and a 600-bed Training Wing. The hospital was entirely devoted to the rehabilitation of psychoneurotics, who, it was hoped, would be able to return to "high grade military duties." The program was not a success. R. Ahrenfeldt, *Psychiatry in the British Army in the Second World War* (London 1958), 149.

60 I have chosen not to identify the individual concerned.

61 Dr Harry Botterell remembers Hanson going off on these expeditions. The U.S. Army's official history speaks of his part in "raids" on the Normandy coast, "Dieppe, the Sicilian Landings, and the front line activity in Tunisia which won him the nickname of the 'Phantom.'" Glass, ed., *Overseas Theatres*, chap. 1.

62 Ibid., chap. 2.

63 Richardson to O.C. Basingstoke, 10 June 43, NAC RG 24, vol. 12631.

64 This term was applied to graduates of the short courses in psychiatry in Canada and the U.K.

65 Interview with Dr Allan Walters, and interviews with Drs Griffin and Richardson.

"A Necessary Nuisance": Social Class and Parental Visiting Rights at Toronto's Hospital for Sick Children 1930–1970

JUDITH YOUNG

Many years before the introduction of insurance schemes, public hospitals in North America admitted a small number of private patients. This practice dated from the late nineteenth century, when modest advances in therapy encouraged hospitals to gain respectability and income by attracting the middle classes. [1] Private patients' benefits included care from a physician of choice and less austere accommodation than was provided on the public wards. Private status conveyed an important additional privilege to families, that of daily access to sick relatives in a time when visiting for most patients was severely limited. [2] Such visiting practices were standard in all hospitals, including those for children. The Hospital for Sick Children Toronto (HSC), Canada's oldest and largest pediatric hospital, will be used to analyse the forms that class distinctions could take in hospitals and the changes that occurred with the advent of hospital insurance and socialized medicine. At HSC discrimination in visiting policies persisted longer than at certain other major pediatric hospitals in Canada, the United States, and Great Britain. [3] This slow change was typical of many hospitals caring for children but atypical of institutions providing leadership in pediatric care.

For decades, when most children entered hospital, they were immediately separated from their parents, who were then restricted to brief weekly visits. Physicians and nurses considered that children settled better in hospital without parents. These ideas and practices were widespread in North America and Britain until the 1950s. Because early hospitals were for the poor, sick children were often removed from unsanitary, destitute homes to what was considered the morally and physically hygienic atmosphere of the hospital.[4] Parents of such children would be unwelcome visitors. Visitors also constituted an infection hazard in the days before antibiotics and immunization. However, from early times the few private patients admitted to special rooms were permitted daily attendance by their parents or nurse.[5]

HSC was primarily a hospital for public patients until hospital insurance introduced semi-private coverage in the 1940s and was expanded in the 1950s. Semi-private status conveyed essentially the same privileges as those afforded private patients, including daily visiting. This was important to parents because HSC appeared slow to acknowledge the results of psychological research that identified the adverse effects of separating children from families.[6] Pediatric institutions such as the Montreal and Winnipeg Children's hospitals promoted visiting for all parents from the late 1940s and early 1950s.[7] But reform at HSC depended on the development of comprehensive health insurance: it was mainly the increase in insured families that led eventually to bed redistribution. Public and private differences gradually disappeared, so that all families were finally granted equal visiting rights, accommodation, and contact with physicians.

EARLY HISTORY OF THE HOSPITAL FOR SICK CHILDREN

The Hospital for Sick Children was founded in 1875 as a charity to serve the poor of Toronto. It was a modest venture, the inspiration of a group of upper-middle-class women (the Ladies Committee). Although many patients received free treatment, parents or friends were encouraged to contribute to the maintenance of the children if they were able. The Ladies Committee was "unwilling to foster pauperism ... [so] strictly enforced the rule of remuneration."[8] Religious fervour influenced the foundation of the hospital but allowed for limited sympathy with the plight of poor families. Drunkenness and failure to live by religious principles were considered to be at the root of the problems of the poor. Such sentiments were expressed in early annual reports, where children were described as living in "an atmosphere of filth, misery and evil, ... [with] sickly and scrofulous constitutions inherited from their drunken and tainted parents."[9]

The wide class distinctions that separated patients from those administering their care influenced subsequent attitudes. Families had little right to question treatment and were mostly grateful for the care their children received in an era when government accepted limited responsibility for the health of its citizens. The social gulf between patients and nurses was not initially wide, but this changed with the development of professional nursing in the late nineteenth century. The "new model nurse" was then recruited from a different social class.[10] The development of nursing at HSC provides illustration of this change. Early HSC nurses were working-class women of good character but without formal training. In 1886 a training school was established that grew in prestige with the growth of the hospital and the acceptance of nursing as a suitable profession for middle-class women.

The tradition of limited visiting at HSC was of long standing and typical of similar institutions. With expansion, children's hospitals became even more restrictive, partly in an attempt to control the spread of infectious diseases. At HSC the first printed regulations, from 1878, state that parents and near relations could visit Wednesdays and Sundays 2–5 P.M.[11] By 1890 families of public patients were restricted to visiting for one hour on Wednesday afternoons. It was hoped that parents would "feel it their duty to conform to these rules, and behave with propriety to the attendants."[12] The hospital was, however, open for public inspection every Saturday. As financing was dependent on donations, those who contributed were encouraged to see how their money was spent. Children were "on show" and expected to be well behaved and friendly.

Local and provincial authorities provided some subsidies that augmented public donations. This became the usual practice in recognition of the "charitable services" rendered by private hospitals.[13] HSC was placed on the provincial "Schedule of Charity Aid" in 1881, and two cents per day was provided for each child.[14] By 1894 the provincial government was paying 36 per cent of the cost of maintenance at thirty-four hospitals, including HSC.[15] Out-patient and in-patient services were free to those "absolutely" unable to pay, providing they had a "circular" from a clergyman or doctor. Payment for indigent patients was provided by municipalities. In 1906, "to protect against imposition," an inspector visited the homes of one hundred patients to "determine if needs were valid." A large number were children of widows or "deserted mothers … living in small, dirty, poorly furnished houses, many in destitute circumstances." The inspector considered that "in all cases drink was the cause of the trouble."[16]

The number of children admitted to HSC increased steadily after the move, in 1892, to a new building on College Street. Although pediatric surgery had progressed, other advances in medical care had little effect on the major problems of pediatric medicine. Malnourished infants living in poverty were at the greatest risk. The increased admission of infants at the turn of the century caused HSC mortality rates to escalate. In 1912, for instance, 65 per cent of infants admitted died, mainly of "intestinal intoxication" and "marasmus."[17] Alan Brown, a young pediatrician, claimed he could halve the death rate in one year and was hired in 1915 as a staff physician.[18] Statistics do show that the infant death-rate declined steadily following Brown's appointment. As physician-in-chief from 1919, Brown was to wield great power and influence at HSC until his retirement in 1951.

From very modest beginnings the Hospital for Sick Children grew steadily in size and in the scope of its services. By 1930 the building on College Street housed between two hundred and three hundred patients. It continued to be primarily a hospital for the poor, and in 1930 most families were unable to pay the daily public rate.[19] Private accommodation was available from 1892, but there is little information regarding its early use. However, regulations in the 1920s clearly outline distinctions in visiting policies between public and private patients. This was the result of a long-standing tradition that granted special privileges to private patients in all hospitals. Visiting at HSC for semi-private patients was daily between the hours of 2 and 4 P.M. Public-ward visiting remained at one hour weekly.[20] This meant that for a three-dollar-a-day semi-private fee, parents could purchase the right to see their children more often. It is not known if parents of private patients were considered less of a hazard in the spread of infection. It is known that they constituted a small minority at the hospital and would have been of a social class similar to the staff's. Thus, the stage was set for long-lasting differences in the treatment of public and private families at HSC.

PUBLIC AND PRIVATE PATIENTS 1930–1945

Little changed in the years 1930 to 1945 to alter the practice of different treatment for public and private families at HSC. The opening of a newly designed private wing in 1935 served to accentuate distinctions in accommodation, but HSC practices regarding special accommodation and daily visiting were essentially no different from practices elsewhere. However, the ratio of public to private patients did gradually change. In the early 1930s most patients were in the public category, and during the Great Depression a high percentage were unable to make any contribution. With greater prosperity and the introduction of Blue Cross insurance by the Ontario Hospital Association in 1941, increasing numbers of families were covered by a prepaid hospital plan. The plan conferred semi-private benefits, which were essentially the privileges afforded private patients. This meant that an increasing number of parents gained closer access to their children despite existing regulations.

The 1930s were years of great hardship for the poor throughout Canada. The Great Depression had its inevitable effect on Toronto and HSC. Intermittently during the early 1930s, 85 per cent of in-patients were on municipal relief orders.[21] The physician-in-chief noted a 50 per cent rise in the use of the out-patient department in two years, with staff physicians giving "free advice to those who could previously pay for expert guidance." There was overcrowding, and there were long hours of waiting. The nurse in charge of the social-service department felt that parents were "apathetic and bitter" and it was hard to obtain their "cooperation."[22]

Despite hard times and reliance on the charity of the hospital, some parents of public patients were dissatisfied enough to remove their children against medical advice. Numbers do not appear to have been recorded, but were significant enough to dismay hospital Superintendent John H. Bower, appointed in 1930. Bower interviewed many of the parents and found them anxious and lacking in information about the hospital. Many could not afford transportation or telephone calls.[23] The majority of "foreign parents were exceedingly nervous," and others removed children "owing to some fancied wrong like not being allowed to visit at any hour."[24] In a unique public-relations move Bower instituted "Parent's Personal Service." A nurse was detailed to follow up cases where parents were known to be dissatisfied. In addition the same nurse maintained contact with out-of-town parents by writing weekly letters providing homely details of the child's condition. In the eyes of Chief Surgeon D.E. Robertson the service did much to promote a "better feeling of goodwill towards the hospital" by the "studied design of paying marked attention to the relatives of patients."[25] Although motivated by concern for the reputation of the hospital, the work of Parent's Personal Service was a humanitarian gesture towards families that remains in existence today.

Government did not accept responsibility at this time for the needs of the poor. By 1936, 36 per cent of the public-ward patients were paying the daily charge of $1.75 on an average weekly income of $18.75 for a family of five. HSC provided this information for the

Ontario government in order to halt a proposed move to discontinue provincial subsidies for paying patients.[26] For critically ill public-ward patients, "special nurses" were provided by the training school at no charge to parents. The Medical Advisory Board set the policy, realizing that extra payment would be "too much of a load" on families.[27]

For further assistance impoverished families relied on the charity of volunteer women's groups. They provided such essential items as extra nourishment, glasses, and diabetic kits, which were distributed by public-health nurses working in the HSC clinics. Annual reports written by the public-health nurses reflect prevailing professional attitudes towards the poor. Nurses deplored the daily confrontation "with the same problems of social maladjustment."[28]

Contemporary accounts of public and private wards at HSC provide illustration of the differences in environment and treatment. William Hawke, later head of neurology and psychiatry, graphically described various public areas of the hospital. In the admitting department a child would be removed from its parent, examined, and sent to the ward. Hawke described the system as something akin to a Chinese laundry, where packages were left and then picked up by the parent when treatment was complete. During the Sunday visiting hour, parents would line up to see the intern or resident on duty; they would of course rarely see a staff doctor.

At one point in his early career Hawke worked close to an area set up in the out-patient department for tonsillectomies on public patients. This he described as an "absolutely incredible situation" and "most thoughtless." Children and parents were lined up outside two rooms, the children "like jayhawks" on the long benches. Sounds of machines pumping (presumably suction apparatus) and children crying could be heard by all.[29] Tonsillectomies on private patients, however, were performed in the main operating room, with children admitted to a private bed for post-operative care.

Most wealthier citizens of Toronto still cared for their sick children at home, with doctor and nurse in attendance. In fact it is considered that many hospitals provided private rooms and wings long before the demand existed.[30] But as techniques, particularly surgery, improved, physicians and surgeons increasingly sought hospital accommodation for their private patients. In 1931 HSC's chief of surgery thought work with "this class of patients" was essential for the hospital and staff.[31] Dr H.J. Cody, president of the University of Toronto, also thought hospital accommodation was needed for the middle class. He felt the poor received the "finest medical and surgical care in Toronto."[32]

In June of 1935 HSC opened a new private wing that followed the tradition of most public hospitals in providing a homelike atmosphere for private patients. The *Toronto Telegram* described the wing as a "fairyland of a hospital." There were frilled pink and white checked gingham drapes, easy chairs, and hooked rugs. Maple furniture was made at the hospital. Beds had carvings of animals and flowers and were covered with candlewick bedspreads. Ferns and bowls of flowers graced the rooms. There was a nursery for infants complete with rocking chairs.[33] The new private facility contrasted sharply with the stark public wards. A photograph from the late 1930s depicts a long ward with no drapes, iron bedsteads, and no chairs or visible toys.[34]

Information about local feeling regarding the public wards at HSC was provided by a patient admitted to the private wing in 1942 and 1944. Apparently local citizens were reluctant to have their children admitted to HSC as there was a stigma attached to being a public patient. Although from a lower-middle-class family of modest means, the patient's mother would not agree to an admission (for an appendectomy) until she had been shown the private facilities by the family's pediatrician.[35]

Visiting for public patients continued to be restricted to one hour on Sundays throughout the period from 1930 to 1945. This was customary in other children's hospitals of the time.[36] It is difficult to know how many hours were permitted for private patients because there are no printed regulations for the 1930s. There are indications, however, that the daily hours were quite liberal: in 1943 the nursing superintendent successfully sought elimination of the morning visiting time.[37] There were also provisions for parents of private patients to stay overnight, though it is unlikely that this was encouraged.[38]

Apart from questions of class and infection control, policies restricting the access of most parents reflected professional views concerning child care in this era. Strict routines were considered a vital aspect of child-rearing, with great attention paid to discipline. Spoiling by undue attention was thought to be harmful, even in the very young.[39] The scientific-feeding movement dictated that infants should be fed at strict intervals and should not be held between feedings. In an article on personality development in the young child, nurses were told that mothers frequently hinder their children from "gaining emotional independence."[40] A period in hospital away from mother was not considered harmful. A physician of this era said that parents were considered a "necessary nuisance,"; presumably, the fewer in number and the closer they were in social class to physicians and nurses, the easier they would be to tolerate.[41]

Professionals continued to adopt an accusing tone when commenting on the social conditions of the poor, the implication being that it was an easy matter for people to improve their status. During the war years many families were affected by the dual problems of absent fathers and working mothers. There were limited social programs to assist the poor with child-rearing. Alan Brown commented unsympathetically on a survey of the socio-economic conditions of three hundred families whose babies were admitted to HSC. He noted that 70 per cent of infants came from a "poor type of home," which accounted for frequent readmissions and increased the "workload of the hospital."[42]

The HSC trustees tried to limit increases in rates, but by 1944 the public rate was up to $3.50 per day for the first week. Families who could not afford to pay required a signed municipal order in their hands to avoid being charged. Families could not elect whether they paid public or semi-private fees. The accounts department was authorized to inquire into family income. If this was considered sufficient, a semi-private rate was enforced. As more treatments became available, paying patients incurred additional costs, such as $5.35 for penicillin and $10 for a blood transfusion.[43]

Most newspaper articles about HSC that appeared in the Toronto press praised the work of the institution highly. *Toronto Telegram* founder John Ross Robertson had been an early benefactor and chairman of the Board of Trustees. The *Telegram* provided much excellent publicity for the hospital. However, by the mid-1940s more critical reports were also appearing in the paper. A 1945 report described a father's concern about his twelve-year-old daughter, admitted for treatment of rheumatic fever. Therapy included the administration of ASA. The father had been refused permission to visit when he arrived in Toronto on a Saturday. When he saw his daughter the next day she was obviously very ill, but no doctor was available to speak to him. Subsequently she was treated for acidosis, due to ASA overdose, but died. The coroner considered the child was "susceptible to the drug" and felt treatment was "competent" given the understaffed wartime conditions. No blame was attached.[44]

The years of the Second World War did see the introduction of Ontario's first group hospitalization plan. HSC Superintendent Bower was a member of a committee set up by the Ontario Hospital Association to do the preparatory work. In 1941 the OHA was authorized by the province of Ontario to operate a hospital-care plan. This became known as the Blue Cross Plan and was qualified for approval by the Blue Cross Commission of the American Hospital Association. As more families were able to take advantage of the insurance, which covered hospitalization costs, the number of public patients at HSC slowly decreased. The increased numbers of semi-private patients had the advantages of daily visiting from parents and choice of staff doctor, though all accommodation was becoming strained in the outdated College Street building.

Apart from some subsidization of hospital beds, direct government payment for health care remained limited to such special situations as treatment of poliomyelitis. A change in government philosophy with regard to responsibility for health and welfare was not to come until the post-war era. In 1945 marked differences remained in the treatment of public and private hospital patients; the Hospital for Sick Children was no exception.

CLASS DISTINCTIONS REMAIN 1946–1955

By 1947, 30 per cent of the patients at HSC were admitted to private or semi-private beds. For public patients the severe restrictions on visiting remained despite increasing evidence from psychologists that such policies could be harmful to children. Access to information from doctors was also a persistent problem for families of public patients. According to long-standing tradition, staff doctors provided free service, but this did not include an obligation to communicate with the family. HSC provides an example of the "elite voluntary hospital" described by Starr. Patients were either poor and received care on the understanding that they were available for teaching purposes, or were rich, and so provided income and bequests. Such hospital were usually old, "had the largest endowments [and] enjoyed the most prestige as centers for medical training and treatment."[45] At HSC the idea that all patients could be considered for teaching purposes did not come until the number of public patients was greatly reduced.

Post-war conditions in Toronto were hard for the less affluent because of a severe housing shortage. Newspapers recorded court cases where parents who had no proper home were charged for failing to remove children from HSC. A navy veteran was told by a magistrate that he had "fallen down as a father" for not being able to provide for his children.[46] A separated mother with seven children was charged under the Ontario Hospital Act with leaving her sick daughter at HSC.[47] The practice of drugging children in order to keep them quiet occurred because some landlords would only accept children if they made no noise. Government grants to day-care

centres, provided in wartime, were reduced and sometimes eliminated as mothers were no longer needed for war work.[48]

At HSC efforts to replace an overcrowded and outdated facility
had been delayed by economic depression and war. A nurse vividly
recalled the situation on the public wards, where she was assigned
to work for three months as an "affiliating" student in 1948. She had
been warned of the chronic shortage of linen and said it was necessary to "kill for a diaper." The infant ward was persistently
overcrowded, and if a nurse were to attend to one baby, several
others would have to be moved. Summer diarrhoea was still prevalent, and deaths were not uncommon.[49]

In 1945 and 1949 highly successful campaigns were conducted to
collect funds for a new Hospital for Sick Children. There was an
embarrassing delay before the first sod could be turned to commence
the new building because a permanent trailer camp, with 150 oc-
cupants, existed on the University Avenue site. The families refused
to move until the city provided a suitable park with facilities. They
held out for five months, turning down an initial offer of accommodation at the Long Branch and Stanley barracks.[50]

A planning committee from HSC had visited other hospitals to get
ideas for the new building. Significantly, they were not influenced
by features giving all parents greater access. In the new hospital the
public infant wards consisted of cubicles with glassed-in viewing
corridors, "so that parents may see but not come into contact with
the patient at any time."[51] On one of the private floors single rooms
were provided for infants. The press emphasized equality of care of
public and private patients in the new hospital. One writer considered the term "public" something of a "misnomer, because there
[would] be no difference in the quality of service and precautionary
methods."[52] Superintendent Bower felt that services were the same,
but the private accommodation was "more attractive and spacious."
He noted that with the increasing number of prepaid insurance
plans, the "sharp distinction" between public and private patients
would gradually lessen.[53] The general public seemed delighted with
the new hospital; during a six-day open house eighty-five thousand
toured the building.

The provincial government continued to pay the hospitalization
expenses of poliomyelitis patients. In the severe epidemic of 1937
this had included a temporary hospital, run by HSC, with stress on
"mental hygiene" and rehabilitation.[54] A further epidemic occurred
in the late 1940s. A post-polio centre was established at Thistletown,
HSC's country branch, where children were encouraged to have a
positive attitude towards their disabilities. The government paid

only for the first hospitalization. A *Globe and Mail* article, describing the treatment program, noted that "children may slump back into crippledom after leaving, due to lack of guidance and money."[55] Patients also required a proven diagnosis in order to benefit from government assistance.

The major Toronto papers continued to provide excellent publicity for HSC. The *Telegram* felt that children received the best medical care, regardless of the parent's capacity to pay.[56] The same paper did, however, report the complaints of an English widow who stated that the hospital held her child until she paid her bill. HSC denied the charges.[57] The appearance of a left-wing press in Toronto led to criticisms of the current hospital system. Articles complained that parents were being interrogated about finances before treatment was provided, with some enduring long waits and discourteous treatment from staff.[58] *Flash Toronto* questioned the "swindle" at HSC, which received donations so that poor children could be treated free. The hospital had sent a bill for $484 to the municipal welfare department, which was now "hounding" a Euclid Avenue couple.[59] The HSC accounts department was accused of "bullying collection tactics," including threats to sue and an attempt to remove one couple from the RCAF Benevolent Fund.[60]

Despite the sensational style of reporting in the left-wing press, complaints do not appear to have been without foundation. In a 1953 report on the admitting and emergency departments, the HSC Medical Advisory Board recommended measures to create better public relations. In 1954 the committee commented on the many complaints from parents of a "mercenary attitude" on the part of the hospital. Collection of money was to be done "more discreetly" in the future.[61]

The increase in semi-private patients led to a bewildering variety of visiting regulations. As private floors became inadequate to house the increasing numbers, semi-private patients were placed on public wards. This meant that on the same ward some children were allowed daily visitors, while others could see their parents only on Sundays. Actual daily visiting hours were more restricted for semi-private patients on public wards than for the same category of patients on a private floor.[62] In the mid-1950s a new category of patient appeared at HSC. Semi-public patients were those whose doctors agreed to accept whatever payment was covered by insurance. They were placed on the public wards and allowed twice-weekly visitors.[63]

Some nursing staff at HSC were distressed by the inequities in visiting rules. They felt differences were unfair and found it impossible to explain to one child why his mother could come only on Sunday while his neighbour had more frequent visitors. A few head nurses tried to gain support among their colleagues for increased public visiting.[64] By this time psychological research had demonstrated the potential harm of separating the child from his or her family.[65] Some hospitals used the results of research to make policy changes; for example, the Winnipeg Children's Hospital eliminated unequal visiting rules in 1947.[66] At HSC, although some staff supported increased visiting, many continued to believe that children were better off in the hospital without parents. However, the few who promoted change managed, despite active opposition, to get public-ward visiting increased to twice weekly by 1955. HSC physicians appeared distinctly unimpressed with the results of psychological research, and consequently there was no general movement for change.

Physician-in-chief Alan Brown, a respected innovator and teacher in pediatrics in Canada, maintained a powerful influence throughout his thirty-six years at HSC. He remained unelected chairman of the medical Advisory Board, which set hospital policies. He did not waver from the opinion that visitors did not belong on the wards of a children's hospital, particularly those in isolation. It is not known what Brown's views were regarding private-ward visiting. It is known that in his own practice he expected parents to follow his instructions implicitly, not to question or to provide suggestions.[67] If parents questioned his treatment, he was unwilling to continue caring for the child. In what became known as "his" hospital, Brown never had to meet the vast majority of parents. Medical rounds on the public wards were conducted with not a parent in sight. His negative attitude to psychiatry was well-known among his colleagues.[68] It is highly unlikely that he would have even read research on the institutionalization of children, as these studies first appeared in psychiatric journals.

Parents had little power to question policies at the hospital. During this era there was also unquestioned faith in professional opinion. A parent recalled that in 1951 she accepted medical advice urging her to allow a two-week "settling-in" period before visiting her four-year-old son in hospital with polio. She expressed great faith in the care provided, despite the pain of short weekly visits during a long hospitalization.[69]

The need to control the spread of infection provided a strong rationale for visiting restrictions, and no parents were allowed on the isolation wards unless a child was critically ill. Scientific procedures to control the spread of infection had gained great credence. Neither nurses nor doctors considered that techniques could be understood or properly carried out by visitors, particularly the un-educated.

SOCIALIZED MEDICINE ASSISTS CHANGE 1956–1970

During the 1950s and 1960s children in hospital were the focus of much continued psychological research.[70] In some pediatric centres radical change followed as visiting hours were liberalized and over-night accommodation provided for mothers. Change in these centres appears to have come because of strong physician leadership and a co-ordinated team approach involving psychologists and social workers. But many hospitals, including HSC, resisted change for many years.

At HSC as elsewhere, nurses and physicians were strongly divided in their acceptance of the new ideas. Nurses who wanted change failed to act together and also were not supported by a hospital-wide philosophy encouraging more humane treatment of families. Many HSC physicians and surgeons remained actively hostile to increased visiting and denied the possibility of emotional trauma except in children who were "emotionally maladjusted before-hand."[71] Perhaps this was the legacy of Alan Brown's teaching. Brown's dominating presence also delayed the transfer of power to administrators who might be more concerned with public relations. At HSC, although visiting regulations were gradually changed, dif-ferences between public and private access remained until the mid-1960s. The expansion of hospital insurance in the 1960s caused HSC to eliminate private wards completely in 1966.

By 1956 only 38 per cent of patients were in the public category. The remainder were either semi-public or semi-private. The private category was practically eliminated by this time (.46 per cent of patients), presumably because families were satisfied with semi-private benefits. Although insurance was providing increasing cov-erage, additional expenses were often a problem. The *Toronto Star* described the plight of a young couple with limited resources who were faced with a possible charge of $250 if they could not provide ten blood donors.[72] The large amount of blood was necessary for heart surgery, a rapidly growing specialty at HSC in the late 1950s. The same couple were concerned about the cost of special nurses. In 1955 the HSC Women's Auxiliary had started a special fund to assist with this type of expenditure.[73]

In 1960 the out-patient department at HSC remained solely for people who could not afford their own doctor, and a means test was necessary in order to get treatment.[74] There was no appointment system, and children and families spent a considerable amount of time waiting. A curious difference in attitude was also apparent in the booking of tonsillectomies. A head nurse from the 1950s recalled that in the summer months it was thought advisable to halt surgery on the semi-private patients during the polio season. Surgery on public patients, however, continued.[75]

The long-standing tradition of unpaid medical service to public patients continued until the introduction of federally funded comprehensive health insurance in 1968. Although most doctors provided service in a spirit of goodwill, the majority at HSC did not see the need to communicate information to parents. A head nurse recalled HSC's chief of surgery reprimanding his resident for spending undue time talking to a parent. He could not understand why time was spent when the patient was "only public."[76]

In 1958 the federal government passed Bill 320, the Hospital Insurance and Diagnostic Services Act, and in the same year the Ontario Hospital Services Commission provided a plan that covered the majority of Ontario citizens for hospital care. By 1962 the idea of distinct semi-private accommodation at HSC was changing, no doubt due to the decrease in public patients. The Medical Advisory Committee approved a reallocation of beds on the medical wards, which resulted in a redistribution of semi-private beds throughout the public wards. The committee felt this would lead to "better care and improved service."[77]

Daily visiting for public patients was finally introduced in 1961 but was restricted to two hours in the afternoon. In 1961 a new HSC administrative director, John Law, invited parents to respond to a questionnaire about their experiences at HSC. Shortly after a directive from Law informed staff that daily visiting was to be instituted for all patients. Private-ward visiting continued to be more generous until 1965, when visiting hours for all patients were changed to 11 A.M. to 8 P.M. As parents became more of a presence in the hospital, concern for public relations led to greater consideration of their views. It was some time, however, before medical staff considered that presence in the hospital entitled parents to an opinion.

In 1966 Law noted that the medical teaching program at HSC, still largely centred around public patients, would need "modifying."[78] A further redistribution of beds completely eliminated separate private wards. This meant that from 1966 teaching occurred throughout the hospital. The elimination of private wards also meant that rooms were assigned on the basis of a child's condition. Semi-private insurance ceased to entitle patients to preferred accommodation at HSC. This was indeed a remarkable change from earlier times.

The final distinction between public and private care related to unpaid physician care. The movement towards a federally initiated health-insurance program had started in the post-war period. Implementation was delayed until the federal government acted on the recommendations of the 1964 Hall Report. The Medical Care Act of 1967, fully implemented throughout Canada by 1972, instituted a shared federal and provincial health-insurance scheme. In Ontario the 1966 Ontario Medical Services Insurance Plan effectively covered those who could not afford insurance. Doctors could now claim fees for patients previously treated free of charge. In 1969 Ontario entered the federal scheme, which ensured comprehensive medical coverage for all citizens. The changes at HSC, which had gradually redressed the inequities between the public and private in-patients, were complete.

CONCLUSION

Between 1930 and 1970 there was a tremendous advance in the treatment of sick children. Antibiotics revolutionized care in all fields of medicine. Immunization changed the pattern of childhood infectious diseases, while surgery made great advances, particularly in treating congenital anomalies. Changing ideas in psycho-social care could also be considered revolutionary. In 1930 children were expected to live through the experience of hospitalization without their families beside them. However, in the 1940s psychological research provided convincing evidence of the harm of separating children from families. But these ideas were slow to influence practice in many institutions.

A few pediatric hospitals in Canada, Britain, and the United States pioneered change in the psychological care of hospitalized children. HSC, well-known for its innovations in medical and surgical care, was slow to implement change in psycho-social care. The reasons appear varied but can be attributed to a conservative medical staff, many of them openly hostile to change, the lack of a co-ordinated hospital-wide philosophy supporting family presence in the hospital, and a divided nursing staff who lacked the power (or will) to institute change until supported by other professionals. This support came with the expansion of psychiatry at HSC and the development of a social-work department. Such departments had been established earlier at children's hospitals that pioneered improved psycho-social care of children.[79]

At HSC comprehensive hospital and medical insurance helped to effect the transition towards equal rights for families. Important among these rights were equal access to the hospital and to communication with medical staff, regardless of social or economic status. Bed redistribution equalized accommodation for all patients. Along with redistribution came the end of two long-standing traditions: the different visiting privileges afforded to "private" families, and the sole use of public patients for medical teaching. Gradually HSC had changed from being primarily a hospital for the poor, with treatment dependent on class, to an institution that provided equal benefits to all patients.

NOTES

All newspaper articles cited are in scrapbooks deposited in the HSC Archives.
1 M.J. Vogel, *The Invention of the Modern Hospital* (Chicago: University of Chicago Press 1980).
2 C.E. Rosenberg, *The Care of Strangers* (New York: Basic Books 1987).
3 J. Young, *Attitudes and Practices towards the Families of Inpatients at the Hospital for Sick Children Toronto from 1935 to 1975*, MScN, University of Toronto 1987.
4 Vogel, *Invention of the Modern Hospital.*
5 H. Medovy, *A Vision Fulfilled: The Story of the Children's Hospital of Winnipeg 1909–1973* (Winnipeg: Pequin Publishers 1979).
6 Young, *Attitudes and Practices.*
7 C.F. James, "The Parent's Point of View," *Canadian Nurse* 52 (1956): 963–6; Medovy, *A Vision Fulfilled.*
8 HSC Archives, *Annual Report 1880.*
9 *Annual Report 1882.*
10 Rosenberg, *Care of Strangers.*
11 *Annual Report 1878.*
12 *Annual Report 1890.*
13 P. Starr, *The Social Transformation of American Medicine* (New York: Basic Books 1982).
14 *Annual Report 1881.*
15 *Annual Report 1894.*
16 *Annual Report 1906.*
17 *Annual Report 1942.*
18 Hospital for Sick Children Medical Alumni, *Dr. Alan Brown* (Toronto: University of Toronto Press 1984).
19 J.S. Crawford, "History of the Hospital for Sick Children 1919–1958," draft copy in the HSC Library.

20 HSC Rules and Regulations signed by Superintendent Watson Swaine (1922–28).

21 Crawford, *History of HSC*.

22 *Annual Report 1930*.

23 In a letter to Miss M. Vesey, 16 July 1966, Alice Boxill gives the history of Parents Personal Service: copy in the possession of Barbara Fox, HSC.

24 *Annual Report 1930*.

25 Ibid.

26 Crawford, *History of HSC*.

27 Hospital for Sick Children, Minutes of the Medical Advisory Board, 13 Mar. 1931, deposited in the HSC Library.

28 *Annual Report 1939*.

29 William Hawke, MD, former medical resident and later head of the Department of Neurology and Psychiatry at HSC, personal communication, 17 Feb. 1987.

30 Rosenberg, *Care of Strangers*.

31 *Annual Report 1931*.

32 *Toronto Telegram*, 16 Oct. 1935.

33 *Toronto Telegram*, 12 June 1935.

34 Max Braithwaite, *Sick Kids: The Story of the Hospital for Sick Children* (Toronto: McClelland & Stewart 1974).

35 Jeannette Carroll, HSC nursing graduate 1954, personal communication, 29 Jan. 1987.

36 Medovy, *A Mission Fulfilled*.

37 MBA Minutes, 14 Oct. 1943.

38 A memo from Superintendent Bower, 28 June 1938, indicates charges for parents of private patients staying overnight: HSC Archives, Accounting File.

39 Alan Brown, *The Normal Child*, 3rd ed. (Toronto: McClelland & Stewart 1932).

40 A.M. Gee, "Personality Development of the Pre-school Child," *Canadian Nurse* 34(1938): 706–9.

41 See n 29.

42 *Annual Report 1942*.

43 Under memo entitled "Terms," dated 1944, HSC Archives, accounting File.

44 *Toronto Telegram*, 15 May 1945.

45 Starr, *Social Transformation*, 171.

46 *Toronto Star*, 18 Dec. 1948.

47 *Toronto Telegram*, 8 Dec. 1949.

48 L. Morris, "Sharp Words from Dr. Brown Regarding the Drugging of Children," *Canadian Tribune*, 7 Mar. 1949.

49 Mary Lou Patrick was training at Toronto General Hospital in 1948 and went to HSC for her pediatric experience: personal communication, 7 Mar. 1987.

50 *Toronto Star*, 30 June 1947.

51 J. Bower, "Serving Sick Children," *Canadian Hospital* 28, no. 2 (1951): 36–43.

52 C. Daniels, "Where No Child Knocks in Vain," *Health* (Nov./Dec. 1949).

53 Bower, "Serving Sick Children."

54 J. Masten, "Nursing Care in Poliomyelitis following the Isolation Period," *Canadian Nurse* 34 (1938): 249–52.

55 M. Fraser, "Post Polio Program at Thistletown," *Globe and Mail*, 27 Nov. 1948.

56 *Toronto Telegram*, 8 Jan. 1948.

57 *Toronto Telegram*, 11 Nov. 1952.

58 *Hush Free Press*, 26 Aug. & 7 Oct. 1950.

59 *Flash Toronto*, 16 Jan. 1954.

60 *Flash Toronto*, 12 Apr. 1954.

61 MAB Minutes, 1953 & 1954.

62 HSC Standing Orders, 1948, HSC Archives. Visiting hours are listed as:

Private – 2:30pm–8pm daily
Public – 2:30pm–3:30pm Sundays
Private and semi-private patients on public wards – 2:30pm–4:30pm and 7:30pm–8:30pm daily.

63 Muriel Richardson, HSC nursing graduate, 1957, personal communication, 8 Mar. 1988.

64 Lucy Ashton, HSC head nurse, 1950s, personal communication, 20 Jan. 1987.

65 J. Bowlby, *Child Care and the Growth of Love* (Harmondsworth: Penguin 1953); J. Robertson, "Some Responses of Young Children to the Loss of Maternal Care," *Nursing Times* 49 (1953): 382–6.

66 Medovy, *A Vision Fulfilled*.

67 Alan Brown, *The Normal Child*, 5th ed. (Toronto: Harlequin 1958).

68 W. Hawke noted it was common knowledge that Alan Brown described psychiatrists as being as "nutty as fruitcakes."

69 Dorothy Leaf, personal communication, 9 Feb. 1987.

70 D.T.A. Vernon, J.M. Foley, R.R. Sipowicz, *The Psychological Responses of Young Children to Hospitalization and Illness* (Springfield, Ill.: Thomas 1965).

71 June Callwood, "How To Help Your Child Prepare for Hospital," *Maclean's*, 28 Apr. 1956.

72 *Toronto Star*, 24 May 1956.

73 *Globe and Mail*, 31 May 1956.

74 MBA Minutes, Feb. 1960.

75 Vorrie Broe was a head nurse on an HSC surgical ward: personal communication, 24 Feb. 1987.

76 Ibid.

77 HSC, Medical Advisory Committee Minutes, May 1962, deposited in the HSC Library.

78 *Pediatric Patter*, Feb. 1966, HSC Archives.

79 Young, *Attitudes and Practices*.

Socialism and Social Insurance in the United States and Canada

STEPHEN J. KUNITZ

PART ONE

In 1906 Werner Sombart wrote a series of articles later republished under the title *Why Is There No Socialism in the United States*?[1] Since than, many have been perplexed by the question. A variety of answers have been offered: the wealth of the country discouraged it, socialism foundering on shoals of roast beef and apple pie; the conservatism of Catholic immigrant workers made them unresponsive to the socialist message; the doctrinaire Marxism of European-born socialists made them unsympathetic to indigenous versions of socialism and made American socialists unwilling to accept the European version; the socialist split with a large part of the labour movement in the 1890s deprived them of a base of mass support; the American tradition of individualism made people unwilling to subordinate themselves to some larger collectivity. It has also been suggested that, in contrast to England, no unified working class emerged in the United States as wave upon wave of immigrants from many different nations swept on to the shores of America, all of whom had to be socialized to the new industrial world.[2]

It is an important question since, as I shall argue, the absence of a socialist party is part of the reason there is no national health insurance in the United States. I shall suggest that American liberalism has worked to make the United States inhospitable to socialism and that when socialist and social democratic movements did develop, they were incorporated into the Democratic party, the result being a lack of an independent electoral base from which to influence policy.

Comparisons with Canada are helpful because the two nations are often considered to be similar in their adherence to classical liberalism. By this I mean the greater importance given to the individual than the collectivity, and the unwillingness of the state to intervene in what are considered the natural laws of the market. Yet Canada has developed national health insurance, albeit not the state medicine feared by many physicians. What accounts for the difference?

A number of writers have observed that the new nations formed by the colonizing efforts of various European nations developed only certain aspects of the mother countries' social and value structures. The United States developed that part of England's social structure that was bourgeois and individualistic. English Canada, as a number of Canadians have commented, retained certain Tory elements as well. Pierre Berton, for example, has said that it was during the War of 1812 that Canadians defined themselves finally and irrevocably as different from Americans. Out of the attempted invasion a Canadian self-consciousness was forged, the key words of which in "Upper Canada were 'loyalty' and 'patriotism' – loyalty to the British way of life as opposed to American 'radical' democracy and republicanism." Berton goes on to observe:

This attitude – that the British way is preferable to the American; that certain sensitive positions are better filled by appointments than by election; that order imposed from above has advantages over grass-roots democracy (for which read "licence" or "anarchy"); that a ruling elite often knows better than the body politic – flourished as a result of an invasion repelled. Out of it, shaped by an emerging nationalism and tempered by rebellion, grew that special form of state paternalism that makes the Canadian way of life significantly different from the more individualistic American way.[3]

Likewise, Quebec retained many features of the French society that had colonized it in the latter part of the eighteenth century but well before the French Revolution. In the case of both Quebec and English Canada, these traditions included a certain degree of conservative collectivism – that is to say, there were many who held the belief that the state had the duty to intervene in economic affairs; that the collectivity took precedence over individuals; and that society was necessarily hierarchical. According to this explanation, socialism in Canada resulted from the blend of liberal egalitarianism and Tory collectivism and could only develop where collectivist traditions already existed. In the case of Canada the development of socialism was also encouraged by the immigration of British socialists, who were not foreign in their new country as European socialists were alleged to be foreign in the United States.[4]

It was, de Tocqueville suggested in the 1830s, the radical individualism and egalitarianism of Americans that made them so ready to join voluntary associations both civil and political: "Whenever, at the head of some new undertaking, you see the Government in France, or a man of rank in England, in the United States you will be sure to find an association."[5] He observed further:

In their political associations, Americans of all conditions, minds, and ages, daily acquire a general taste for association, and grow accustomed to the use of it. There they meet together in large numbers, they converse, they listen to each other, and they are mutually stimulated to all sorts of undertakings. They afterwards transfer to civil life the notions they have acquired, and make them subservient to a thousand purposes. Thus it is by the enjoyment of a dangerous freedom that the Americans learn the art of rendering the dangers of freedom less formidable.

If a certain moment in the existence of a nation be selected, it is easy to prove that political associations perturb the State, and paralyse productive industry; but take the whole life of a people, and it may perhaps be easy to demonstrate that freedom of association in political matters is favourable to the prosperity and even to the tranquillity of the community.[6]

The political associations de Tocqueville observed were parties, perhaps the first that were truly modern in character. They were a product of individualism and the lack of established hierarchies, for only such organizations could shape a power-base out of a mass electorate. Parties thus became a force for stability in a society in which individualism was the dominant value and population growth and diversity an overwhelming fact of political life. Indeed, it was largely through the Democratic party that immigrants from all across Europe were incorporated into American society.

During much of the nineteenth century and for the first several decades of the present century, the immigrants' route was often by way of local political machines and bosses, an institution peculiar to the United States. These machines were closely linked both to municipal politics and to the Democratic party. New York's Tammany Hall was a typical operation: in return for votes and the opportunities for graft both honest and dishonest, Tammany helped to ease the adjustment of Irish newcomers to America. Contemporary defenders of Tammany emphasized its importance in socializing immigrants to a new city and way of life. Even critics of the system acknowledge that the political bosses understood the immigrants' needs better than the businessmen who were often associated with reform administrations. The point is, however, that Tammany and organizations like it lacked an expansive vision of the possibilities of American life. As Arthur Mann has written, "No matter who ran them, the big-city machines were designed and fueled to win elections and divide the spoils. That takes cunning, industry, sobriety, and organizational know-how, but it requires no social vision. Tammany failed to use, and also misused and abused, the immense power it won because its leaders could not envision a more just and more beautiful city than the mean and ugly neighborhoods in which they grew to manhood."[7]

Tammany's was not the only vision available to the Irish-American community. There was the conservatism of the Catholic Church and, of particular interest here, the social radicalism of the Knights of Labor and some branches of the Land League. These latter movements receded in the 1880s. Presumably similar divisions existed within other immigrant groups, but the important point is that it was the Democratic party that absorbed them. On the one hand, it often absorbed the most radical immigrants – socialists and communists from the Old World – and with them, "labor reform positions on the local level."[8] On the other, the municipal bosses also became part of the Democrats' infrastructure, bringing forward an interest-group agenda that lacked a sense of justice for the broader community. This pattern persists today, as the Democratic party assimilates reformers of the left, submerging their ideology in the mainstream of interest-group politics. And it is in this context that the so-far unsuccessful quest for national health insurance in the United States may be traced.

PART TWO

The connection between pressure for social insurance and socialism – or the fear of socialism – has been obvious for a century, ever since Bismarck's reforms, which were aimed at drawing the teeth of the German socialists.[9] Although Britain was the birthplace of classical liberalism, British social insurance developed relatively early and under the influence of the German experience.[10] Indeed, British society was characterized not by liberalism but by a complex mix of Toryism, liberalism, and working-class self-consciousness. There are even those who claim that the enterpreneurial spirit of liberal individualism was never completely assimilated to British values, the failure contributing largely to Britain's present decline.[11] However that may be, it is certainly true that social insurance was not resisted as vigorously in Britain as in the United States in the first decade or two of this century, and was even found acceptable by many members of the British business community.[12] Certainly the appeal to national efficiency was far more effective in Great Britain after the poor showing of her troops in the Boer War than was the same appeal in the United States.

The appeal to efficiency in the United States served a variety of purposes for the reformers who favoured national health insurance.[13] Among the most important was that it became the ideology of those aspiring to professionalize a number of service occupations. What we required, they believed, was the giving up of the belief in laissez-faire and the development of a bureaucratically organized state staffed by experts who could be in control of the large variety of social problems. Social insurance, including national health insurance, was one of the solutions the reformers offered for the social atomization that, they believed, followed as night follows day the firm adherence to classical liberalism. Theirs was clearly a collectivist view of society, and though only a small number of them were socialists, they were able before the First World War to collaborate with socialists in agitating for this reform. Included in their number were a few business leaders and physicians. They were opposed by Samuel Gompers of the American Federation of Labor and by many business leaders, including those in commercial insurance companies. The appeal to national efficiency that had been so effective in England did not strike a responsive chord in the United States. Growing resistance from the rank and file of the American Medical Association, coupled with the hardships of the First World War, the "red scare" that followed, and the seeming prosperity of the 1920s, put an effective end to the first campaign for social insurance.

The health-insurance campaign began again in the late 1920s, when a number of the reformers from the first campaign, joined by some new recruits and supported by eight private foundations, launched a five-year study that developed into the Committee of the Costs of Medical Care.[14] The committee had its origin in the efforts of several leaders of the AMA who were favourably disposed to national health insurance to study more thoroughly the problem of paying for medical care. This represented a change of focus from the first campaign, which had been directed at reimbursing the worker for time lost from the job as a result of sickness. By the 1920s, as medical care became increasingly hospital-based and thus increasingly expensive, attention shifted to paying for services.[15] In

1926 a committee was formed that included non-physicians and called itself the Committee on the Cost of Medical Care (later to be changed to Costs). Initial support was received from the Twentieth Century Fund, founded by the well-known progressive owner of a large Boston department store, Edward Filene. Filene had been active in the American Association for Labor Legislation, the reformist organization that before the First World War had led the fight for social insurance. By the end of the five-year study the committee consisted of forty-eight members, and funding had been received from eight private foundations.

It is not absolutely clear why private foundations became involved in the study of medical care in the 1920s. The Twentieth Century Fund perhaps primarily reflected Edward Filene's long-standing interest in progressive labour legislation. The Russell Sage Foundation, the Milbank Memorial Fund, the New York Foundation, and the Josiah Macy Jr Foundation had histories of involvement in various social-reform activities. The Carnegie Corporation had been concerned with rationalization of the educational system, from primary to professional school, as well as support for libraries, the arts, and so on. The Julius Rosenwald Fund, established by the president of Sears, Roebuck, had a history of support for the education of blacks, the improvement of race relations, and the provision of medical care. The Rockefeller Foundation was well known for its support of public health and basic biomedical research.[16]

Much has been written about private foundations and the goals of social and political stability they sought to achieve, particularly that of making the world safe for capitalism.[17] This is not a topic I shall pursue here. Except for the Rockefeller philanthropies, foundation archives have not been easily accessible to researchers, so it is not really possible to know what determined the policies they pursued. Official histories are not especially helpful in this regard. Moreover, even among the foundations that supported the CCMC there seem to have been major differences in emphasis. Finally, no matter what the original intent of benefactors and their advisers, over time foundation officers may have changed the missions of their organizations. Not so long ago Henry Ford II resigned from the board of the Ford Foundation claiming that its executives and staff had forgotten that it was capitalism that had made their activities possible in the first place.

In general, foundations were the creations of men who had made fortunes by managerial innovations. Filene and Rosenwald had done in marketing and distribution what Carnegie and Rockefeller had done in extraction and manufacturing. That is to say, new techniques of managerial efficiency and control – what has been called "the visible hand"[18] – had replaced the invisible hand of the market. And just as the market was no longer to be left to operate freely, neither could people-processing systems, of which medical care was a prime example. As in the earlier campaign for social insurance, so behind the support of the CCMC, I believe, was the expectation that examination of the data by experts would lead to rational solutions with which all men would agree.

If that was the hope, it was not realized. The final report of the CCMC was published in 1932, three years after the start of the Great Depression and just as the Democrats were entering the White House.[19] The committee was split, and majority and minority reports were issued, along with several dissenting statements by individual committee members. The majority favoured voluntary prepaid health insurance and salaried physicians only in rural or poor areas. This recommendation was clearly influenced by the municipal-doctor system in Saskatchewan, which had been the subject of an early CCMC report by C. Rufus Rorem.[20]

The majority, which included academic physicians, public representatives, and social scientists, could scarcely have been considered revolutionary even fifty years ago. They were evidently so regarded by the minority (composed primarily of representatives of the AMA), however, and by much of the medical and lay press, which favoured a continuation of fee-for-service private practice without the intervention of any form of insurance. Morris Fishbein, editor of the *Journal of the American Medical Association*, wrote of the majority and minority reports: "These two reports represent ... the difference between incitement to revolution and a desire for gradual evolution based on analysis and study ... The alignment is clear – on one side the forces representing the great foundations, public health officialdom, social theory – even socialism and communism – inciting to revolution; on the other side, the organized medical profession of this country urging an orderly evolution guided by controlled experimentation which will observe the principles which have been found through the centuries to be necessary to the sound practice of medicine."[21]

Even among the majority there was not real unanimity. The final recommendation did not include compulsory national health insurance for all, only voluntary group insurance. A number of the members of the committee and staff had favoured a much stronger position in respect of compulsory insurance but compromised with those favouring voluntarism in the interests of presenting a united front to those opposed to any form of insurance whatever. After the CCMC finished its work, several of these individuals continued to

press for compulsory national health insurance, among them
Michael Davis, director of Medical Services of the Rosenwald Fund,
and Edgar Sydenstricker, director of Research, and I.S. Falk, research associate, of the Milbank Memorial Fund. [22] Shortly thereafter
the latter two became respectively director and staff assistant of the
Technical Committee on Medical Care of the Cabinet-level Committee on Economic Security established by newly elected President
Roosevelt to develop plans for what was to become the Social Security Bill. [23]

Both Sidenstricker and Falk were active in urging inclusion of
compulsory national health insurance in·the Social Security Bill as
it was being prepared in 1934 and 1935. The powerful AMA lobby
and congressional resistance convinced the president and his Cab-
inet that such a step would threaten the chances of the entire bill,
of which unemployment insurance and old-age benefits were the
most important features. Thus by 1935 it had been decided not to
include such a provision: "Compulsory health insurance failed in
the Committee on Economic Security for two related reasons. The
immediate cause was the superiority of the political tactics and strategy of the anti-insurance forces. The more fundamental cause was
the lack of any broadly based public feeling that medical care needed
a reform as drastic as compulsory insurance seemed to be." [24]

The constitutionality of the Social Security Act was in doubt until
a Supreme Court decision in 1937. After that, consideration turned
to amending and improving it, and once again efforts were made
to include compulsory insurance. The amendments that were passed
in 1939, however, included on the one hand provisions for extending
benefits to survivors of beneficiaries while on the other reducing the
number of people eligible to be beneficiaries. [25] Proposed amendments to the Social Security Act that covered health insurance were
included in the Wagner Bill of 1939. The bill gave the states the right
to participate or not in each of a number of programs, all of which
were basically aimed at providing relief for the indigent rather than
universal coverage. There was, however, the possibility that programs could later be expanded to other segments of the population.
Despite dilution of the provisions the reformers had hoped for, the
Wagner Bill was defeated by a combination of divisiveness among
the pro-insurance group, active lobbying by the AMA, an increasingly conservative Congress, lack of support from the president,
whose attention was increasingly being drawn to international affairs, and lack of widespread public support.

There were several reasons for the lack of public support. First,
increasingly voluntary hospitalization insurance was developing.
The most notable program was Blue Cross, sponsored by the hospital

associations in response to the deficits and cash-flow problems incurred by general hospitals during the Depression. Indeed, C. Rufus Rorem, one of the CCMC staff, had been supported by the Rosenwald Fund to help establish Blue Cross in the mid-1930s. As voluntary insurance programs expanded, growing but still small numbers of the employed enrolled, thus draining off some potential supporters of compulsory national insurance. Moreover, the AMA began to soften its opposition in principle to insurance and by the late 1930s had accepted its inevitability. Opposition to national insurance remained firm, however, voluntary programs being the only ones found acceptable.

Second, organized labour, currently the single most important advocate of national health insurance, was only emerging as an important political force during the 1930s. As already noted, Samuel Gompers had for a long time been opposed to all forms of state insurance. The reason for his opposition and that of the AFL leaders who followed him in the late 1920s and early 1930s was that if benefits were not tied to union membership, there would be one less reason for workers to remain loyal to their unions.

The posture of labour leaders with respect to national health insurance began to change in the 1930s for several related reasons. The AFL had organized primarily along craft lines. Industry-wide unons were unusual in the early decades of the century. Even by the early 1930s, when mass production had become an established fact of industrial life, the AFL leadership continued to reflect its origins by generally refusing to organize along other than craft lines. Passage of the National Industrial Recovery Act in 1933 and the Wagner (National Labor Relations) Act in 1935, by forbidding employers to prohibit unionization and requiring them to bargain only with the union elected to represent their workers, gave a great impetus to unionizing. It was in this context that John L. Lewis, Sidney Hillman, and other AFL leaders broke away from the parent organization to found the Congress of Industrial Organization (CIO).[26] Their success in organizing mass-production industries – and the success of the AFL in doing the same when spurred by competition from the CIO – resulted in an increase of union membership in the course of the 1930s from perhaps three million to eight million.[27]

Not only did union membership increase, but the new unions tended to be more left-wing politically than the older ones. Radicals had been active in the American labour movement since the 1880s but had never dominated it. Nor did they dominate it in the 1930s. Undoubtedly, however, their influence increased at this time for several reasons. First, the Depression caused many workers to question the capitalist system. Second, the encouragement the new federal legislation provided unionization allowed disciplined and ideologically sophisticated organizers, very often Communist party members, access to previously unorganized workers in mass-production industries. Third, the personal courage, dedication, and organizational skills of many left-wing labour leaders inspired loyalty among many rank-and-file members.[28]

It was in the course of this transition from relatively small, conservative, craft-dominated unions in the early 1930s to large, politically active, industrial, left-wing unions by the late 1930s that attitudes towards social insurance on the part of the labour leadership began to change, including attitudes towards national health insurance. Labour's only representative on the Committee on the Costs of Medical Care had been John Frey, a leader of the AFL. Labour was so invisible that Morris Fishbein did not even include it among the groups he chose to attack in his vitriolic editorial cited above. Frey was not one of those committee members who believed in compulsory national health insurance. Several editorials appeared in the *American Federationist* in 1932 and 1933 supporting the majority recommendations of the CCMC; none advocated anything wider in scope. But by the time the Wagner Bill of 1939 was under consideration, labour was well represented among its advocates.[29] What accounts for the change?

In 1934 and 1935 the old leadership still held sway. The split that would lead to the large organizing drives of the industrial unions was still in the future, made possible by legislation passed at just the time the Social Security Bill was being drafted. Thus there was no voice representing the millions of still unorganized workers to be raised in favour of national health insurance in the early 1930s.

With the official recognition of organized labour's right to represent workers, one of the reasons for opposing social insurance disappeared. If unions were now relatively more secure as the duly elected representatives of workers in many industries, then it was less crucial that the workers' loyalty to the union be held by benefits administered only through the union. Further, the disaster of the Depression must have made it obvious that unions alone could not protect their members during those times when large numbers of them were unemployed. Only the federal government was big enough to do that.

Thus the expansion of membership along industrial lines, the recruitment of more radical workers, and the more secure place of unions all worked to encourage labour's increasing support for national health insurance. But the time when such legislation might have passed was lost in 1938 as a result of the election of the most conservative congress of the New Deal period,[30] the distraction provided by events in Europe, continued divisiveness among the pro-insurance forces, and continued opposition by the AMA.[31]

The growth of left-wing industrial unionism did not mean the emergence of a socialist third party. Organized labour increasingly became integrated into the Democratic party, perhaps as the locus of a social democratic movement, as Michael Harrington has suggested.[32] In a series of lectures to the International Ladies' Garment Workers' Union in 1943–45, University of Wisconsin economist Selig Perlman explained the situation as follows:

It is but natural that Europeans should be puzzled when they try to figure out what the American political party is. It does not seem to conform to any particular model of political party that they as Europeans are accustomed to. It seems very much like a crazy quilt.

Take the Democratic party with its very heterogeneous composition; it does look like a crazy quilt. Altogether different groups seem to unite on Election Day on the national candidates but on the day after the election those groups may be and often are at each other's throats. They have very little in common. In fact, they are quite antagonistic to each other. And that creates the impression of the instability of this typical American political party ...

Such is the structure of politics in the United States. I know that to many of us this picture is in some way distasteful, perhaps very much so. We would like to have a political party that would express fully our ethical commitments and our social objectives. But I am sorry to say – and I have to say it because it is my conviction – that I believe that such a realignment in our political life would really operate to enthrone the conservatives in power forever. This is basically a very conservative country, it is a country in which the labor movement lives in a rather hostile environment, hostile either actually or potentially. This is why I do not believe in this kind of clearcut, independent political action. I fear the result. I fear that the result would be to render the attainment of our social and ethical objectives practically impossible. Whether we like it or not, the kind of political action that we are obliged to follow is the method of collective bargaining in politics, pressure politics.[33]

Radical farm groups experienced something similar. It is not necessary to go into this in any detail save to make one point. There had been radical farmers' groups before the 1930s, the most significant for my purpose being the Non-Partisan League in the northern midwest, especially among the wheat farmers in North Dakota, just across the border from Saskatchewan. The NPL was not precisely the same as the Co-operative Commonwealth Federation (CCF) in Saskatchewan, though they did have much in common. As Seymour Lipset has observed: "The radicalism and strength of the NPL, which remained a faction of the Republican Party, waned after economic prosperity began to return and the farmers received their immediate economic objectives of a guaranteed parity price and crop insurance from the federal government."[34] That is to say, farmers too became an interest group represented within the two major parties – as well as a bloc dealing autonomously with the federal government.[35]

Contrast with this the situation in Canada:

The Liberal-CCF relationship in 1943–45 is only the sharpest and clearest instance of the permanent interdependence forced upon each by the presence of the other, a relationship which one student describes as "antagonistic symbiosis." The Liberals depend on the CCF-NDP for innovations; the CCF-NDP depend upon the Liberals for implementation of the innovations. When the left is weak, as before and after the Second World War, the centre party moves right to deal with the Conservative challenge; when the left is strengthened, as during the war and after the formation of the NDP, the centre moves left to deal with that challenge ...

Socialism was not powerless, so there was no New Deal. There was no New Deal, so socialism grew more powerful. Socialism grew more powerful, so King reacted with "A New Social Order for Canada."[36]

Not all Canadian scholars agree with this explanation. Some claim that the CCF had no impact on Liberal policies in the 1940s.[37] None the less, it is striking that a significant, albeit minority socialist party has survived in Canada, has at times controlled provincial governments, and has even knocked on the doors of national power. Nothing similar has happened in the United States.

Certainly with respect to national health insurance it is significant that the socialist government of Saskatchewan was the first in North America to attempt social insurance, starting with universal, publicly administered hospital coverage in 1947 and followed by more complete protection in the late 1950s and early 1960s.[38] A detailed history of health care in Saskatchewan is unnecessary here. The key point is that pioneering policies pursued in Saskatchewan had a considerable impact nationally.[39] Despite the turmoil of the doctors' strike of 1962, for instance, the essentials of Saskatchewan's plan for physician reimbursement were adopted nation-wide several years later.[40] Despite business opposition, as well as Conservative opposition at the provincial level, at the federal level Conservatives were virtually unanimous in their support of both hospital insurance in the 1950s and physician reimbursement plans in 1976–78,[41] a unanimity made possible by the party discipline that can be enforced in parliamentary systems such as Canada's.

This supports my view that Canadians at virtually all points on the political spectrum have a more collectivist orientation towards society and the role of government than do Americans. More than Americans, Canadians regard as legitimate government's claim to protect the well-being of all citizens for the national good. As the case of conservative collectivists indicates, this is not incompatible with an acceptance of inequality of socio-economic status; it is indeed an example of *noblesse oblige*. That is to say, the presence of a viable socialist party in Canada does not mean that Canada is not a capitalist country. It suggests, however, that socialism is viewed as legitimate by significant sections of the public and that even many non-socialists share with them a vision of society as a collectivity with responsibility for the well-being of its members. This is not the same as saying that socialism is merely and intermittently tolerated, which is I think more nearly the case in the United States. The same orientation that makes socialism legitimate makes social insurance widely acceptable as well.

An indication of the legitimacy of socialism in Canada is the relative absence of virulent red-baiting as compared with several such episodes in America's past. Indeed, two of the administrators of Saskatchewan's health program in the late 1940s were American believers in socialized medicine who presumably left their own country for a more hospitable climate.[42] And Saskatchewan's original health-care plan was based upon the report of a committee chaired by Johns Hopkins professor Henry Sigerist, who left the United States for Switzerland shortly after the Second World War when the political climate became increasingly unfriendly.

These episodes are symbolic of the problems American social-democratic reformers faced when attempting to develop national health insurance. If Canadian Liberals were forced to respond to a strong left-wing movement by developing national health insurance, American social-democratic reformers during the same period were forced to look to their right and tailor their proposals to the contours of a much different body politic.

PART THREE

After the defeat of President Truman's insurance plan in 1949, pro-insurance reformers began to think in much more modest terms than coverage for the entire population. They settled upon the elderly recipients of social-security benefits as the most likely group.[43] This group could not be blamed for being old and having high rates of acute and chronic illnesses. Moreover, it was considered that, as social-security beneficiaries, they had in a sense earned the right to protection by having contributed to the fund during their working years. To attack socialized medicine was one thing; to attack the deserving elderly quite another, particularly when health-care costs were being paid by working children.

Already in the late 1930s the AMA had begun to approve of some kinds of private insurance. Thus by the 1950s it was not enough simply to oppose government insurance; alternative proposals were necessary. The differences between various bills have been described elsewhere.[44] What I want to point out is the very different assumptions underlying them.

As I have already noted, the reformers chose elderly social-security recipients because they were believed to have rights to services by virtue of having contributed during their working lives. The reformers continued to believe that simply as citizens people were entitled to services without having to prove need, but the elderly represented a conscious change in strategy: categorial programs were a foot in the door.

The opponents of reform believed not in universal entitlement but in individual responsibility. For those who, for whatever reason, could not care for themselves, some form of charitable help had to be provided, analogous to physicians' sliding-fee schedules. This would, of course, require a means test, and to minimize federal intervention the program would have to be under the control of state governments. Once need had been proved according to local criteria, coverage would in fact be much more complete than was provided for in the reformers' proposals.

During the Eisenhower years there was no chance that the reformers' bill would be passed, though it is worth observing that, as a compromise with pro-insurance reformers, increasing amounts of money each year were spent on federal support of biomedical research, with profound consequences for schools of medicine, medical education, and medical care.[45] Even during President Kennedy's term of office, liberal Democrats did not command enough votes for passage of Medicare. Only as a result of the Democratic landslide in 1964 that brought President Johnson to the White House did passage became inevitable. In an ingenious legislative stroke, two bills – the reform bill covering social-security recipients and the conservative bill covering the poor – were combined into Medicare and

Medicaid. The first was based upon the reformers' belief in universal entitlement, the second upon their opponents' belief in individual responsibility, local control, and the need for means testing.

Medicare and Medicaid had profound consequences. With respect to cost, numerous studies showed that health care became increasingly expensive after passage because physicians and hospitals were reimbursed on a fee-for-service basis at prevailing customary rates. Indeed, once physicians understood how much they would benefit from the legislation, they became much more positive in their attitudes towards it.[46] As costs continued to increase, and particularly after the economic downturn beginning in the early 1970s, the Republican administration became increasingly concerned with the issue of cost containment. It was in this context that health-maintenance organizations modelled upon the Kaiser-Permanente prepaid plans and previously anathematized by the AMA came to be seen as a panacea. It was also in this context that there was increasing attention devoted to matters of unhealthy "lifestyles" and self-care – victim-blaming, as it was called by its critics.

Because, however, Medicare and Medicaid had institutionalized the government's involvement in health care in a new and massive way, there was no turning back. Instead, further discussions of national health insurance, stimulated largely by Walter Reuther and the formation of the Committee of One Hundred, were based upon the left's efforts to expand and rationalize the government's health-care programs and the right's efforts to control expansion and contain costs while directing those profits that were to be made to the private sector. Thus in the early 1970s several bills were debated in Congress.

The administration's national health-insurance proposal included three components: "The employee health care insurance plan for working families, the assisted health care insurance plan for the poor, and the federal health care insurance plan to replace Medicare for the elderly." Major provisions of the proposal are accessible elsewhere.[47] It is enough to point out here simply that employees were to be covered by policies with private insurance companies, resulting in enormous profits to that industry; the program for the poor was to continue to be administered by the states, which would have considerable discretion regarding reimbursement levels; and physicians would have the option of being full or associate participating providers, the latter category permitting the possibility of charging fees above those established by the state in which they practised.

There were a number of other bills proposed by the AMA, the American Hospital Association, and the health-insurance industry.

Virtually all would have left some citizens uncovered, and all would have meant substantial income for private insurance companies and the continuance of prevailing fees for physicians.

At the other end of the ideological spectrum was the Kennedy-Griffith Health Security Bill, supported by the AFL-CIO as well as the minuscule Socialist party. This was a universal plan involving only the federal government and based upon the assumption that health care is the right of all. The involvement of state agencies and private insurance companies was to be minimal. Budgeting was to be prospective, based upon the previous year's expenditures.[48]

In the event, none of these bills was passed into law. By the late 1960s the era in American politics that had begun with the New Deal was ending. A rightward shift had occurred that, combined with the economic decline starting in the early 1970s, made it unlikely that any national health-insurance scheme would be adopted in the 1970s and 1980s. I can only suggest here some of the reasons for this shift.[49]

First, post-war prosperity and federal support of road-building and home ownership had allowed many ethnic Americans to join the middle class and move to the suburbs. They were replaced in many urban neighbourhoods by southern blacks, Puerto Ricans, and others.

Second, as the Democratic party embraced blacks and other minority groups during the heady days of the New Frontier and the Great Society, many of its traditional supporters – working- and middle-class whites in the urban north and rural south – shifted to the Republicans, often by way of George Wallace's third party. Indeed, in the 1980 presidential election 43 per cent of voters from union households voted for Ronald Reagan despite the bulk of formal union endorsement of Jimmy Carter.[50]

Third, the growing economy of the Sun Belt attracted an increasing number of working- and newly middle-class whites. The result was that many of these formerly Democratic states became firmly Republican, with enough electoral votes largely to determine presidential elections. Moreover, these massive population shifts worked a measurable change in the composition of the Congress, where the consequences with respect to health-care policy have been readily discernible.[51] It must be added, however, that participation in recent elections has been remarkably low, on the order of 50 per cent of eligible voters casting ballots in presidential races. If participation were to increase for some reason, such as the catastrophic economic collapse that occurred during the Depression of the 1930s, the results would not be at all certain. It is possible that non-voters are primarily

the traditional supporters of the Democratic party, and their participation could make a profound difference in the future.

PART FOUR

I observed in passing that efforts at cost containment had resulted
in the paradox of a Republican administration's turning to prepaid
health-care plans, previously anathematized as socialist. Health-
maintenance organizations, as such organizations are called, are
multi-specialty groups of physicians that provide subscribers all care
for which they have contracted, for an agreed price. Since the group
is at risk if costs of care exceed income, the incentive is to do as little
as possible, just the reverse of the incentives under fee-for-service
methods of reimbursement. To accuse such groups of practising
"socialized medicine," as the AMA did until only recently, is inaccurate. Many are now owned by for-profit corporations for which
physicians work as employees (often without financial incentives to
reduce expenditures), an oft-cited example of the proletarianization
of a once-free profession. No matter what the ownership, however,
the requirement is to cut costs by doing as little as possible and by
recruiting healthy enrollees ("selecting against adverse risk," as it is
euphemistically known). Thus these groups are primarily for the
employed. Attempts at enrolling the poor (for example, Medicaid
recipients) have not been notably successful.

Similar principles of managing use of hospital services have been
extended by the federal government to Medicare patients through
so-called diagnosis-related groups (DRGs). The result have been un-
happiness among physicians, lack of adequate care for the uninsured
(numbering perhaps thirty-five million to forty million), and bureaucratic barriers to care for many people with coverage. That is to
say, the competitive solution to the problem of providing care within
the constraints of limited budgets has not proved effective. In contrast, in 1984 the Canadian Liberal federal government imposed
penalties on provinces that allowed extra billing by doctors or charging of user fees by acute-care hospitals. The Conservative party
unanimously supported the legislation (the Canada Health Act) and
implemented it when they won a large majority in the House of
Commons later that same year.

It has been argued by some that the massive budget deficits that
accumulated during the Reagan years were engineered intentionally
to make it impossible for any subsequent administration to reinsti-
tute the welfare spending of the Great Society, including efforts at
creating national health insurance. Whether intended or not, a con-

sequence of large federal deficits has been to make universal coverage under national health insurance less likely than some had believed possible even a decade ago.[52] Whether the United States will ever achieve such a form of care is of course impossible to predict. It seems unlikely, however, at least in the near future, because the forces that have made it possible elsewhere are here submerged as simply one among many interest groups.

NOTES

I am grateful to William Bluhm, Theodore Brown, David Coburn, Frederick Glaser, Stephen Mick, C. David Naylor, and Ernest Saward for comments.

1 W. Sombart, *Why Is There No Socialism in the United States?* (London: Macmillan 1976).

2 H.G. Gutman, *Work, Culture, and Society in Industrializing America* (New York: Alfred A. Knopf 1976).

3 Pierre Berton, *The Invasion of Canada* (Toronto: McClelland and Stewart 1980), 313–14. Of scholarly interest here is the volume edited by Sydney F. Wise, *Canada Views the United States: Nineteenth-Century Political Attitudes* (Seattle: University of Washington Press 1967). Among the pertinent essays on Canadian attitudes is Wise's own contribution, "Colonial Attitudes from the Era of the War of 1812 to the Rebellions of 1837," 16–43.

4 G. Horowitz, *Canadian Labour in Politics* (Toronto: University of Toronto Press 1968), chap. 1. That Canadian society has remained more hierarchical – more "English," in fact – than American is widely agreed. There is no agreement concerning the causes. See, for instance, D. Harrison, *The Limits of Liberalism: The Making of Canadian Sociology* (Montreal: Black Rose Books 1981). My own sympathies incline me towards the argument that continued dependence upon England was favoured by merchant capitalists who benefited by the special trading relationship. How this relationship may in turn be related both to differences in political culture among classes and regions of Canada and to the domination of Canadian industry by American corporations has not to my knowledge been well worked out. This topic is beyond the bounds of this paper. It is one that Canadian scholars seem increasingly to be pursuing.

5 Alexis de Tocqueville, *Democracy in America* (New York: Schocken Books 1961), vol. ii, book ii, chap. 5.

6 Ibid., chap. 7.

7 A. Mann, "Introduction," in W.L. Riordon, *Plunkitt of Tammany Hall* (New York: E.P. Dutton 1963), xx–xxi.

8 E. Foner, "Class, ethnicity, and radicalism in the Gilded Age: the Land-League and Irish-America," *Marxist Perspectives* (Summer: 1978): 46.

9 H.E. Sigerist, "From Bismarck to Beveridge: Development and Trends in Social Security Legislation," *Bulletin of the History of Medicine* 13(1943): 365–88.

10 B.B. Gilbert, *The Evolution of National Insurance in Great Britain: The Origins of the Welfare State* (London: Michael Joseph 1966).

11 M.J. Wiener, *English Culture and the Decline of the Industrial Spirit, 1850–1980* (Cambridge: Cambridge University Press 1981).

12 R. Hay, "Employers and Social Policy in Britain: The Evolution of Welfare Legislation, 1905–14," *Social History*, no. 4 (1977): 435–55.

13 S.J. Kunitz, "Efficiency and Reform in the Financing and Organization of American Medicine in the Progressive Era," *Bulletin of the History of Medicine* 55 (1981): 497–515.

14 F.A. Walker, "Americanism versus Sovietism: A Study of the Reaction to the Committee on the Costs of Medical Care," *Bulletin of the History of Medicine* 53 (1979): 489–504.

15 P. Starr, "Transformation in Defeat: The Changing Objectives of National Health Insurance, 1915–1980," *American Journal of Public Health* 72 (1982): 78–88.

16 J. Ettling, *The Germ of Laziness* (Cambridge: Harvard University Press 1981).

17 E.R. Brown, *Rockefeller Medicine Men* (Berkeley: University of California Press 1979). H.S. Berliner, "A Larger Perspective on the Flexner Report," *International Journal of Health Services* 5 (1975): 573–92, and "New Light on the Flexner Report: Notes on the AMA-Carnegie Foundation Background," *Bulletin of the History of Medicine* 51 (1977): 603–9.

18 A.D. Chandler, Jr, *The Visible Hand: The Managerial Revolution in American Business* (Cambridge: Harvard University Press 1977).

19 Committee on the Costs of Medical Care, *Medical Care for the American People* (Chicago: University of Chicago Press 1932).

20 C.R. Rorem, *The "Municipal Doctor" System in Rural Saskatchewan.* (Chicago: University of Chicago Press 1931).

21 Quoted in D.S. Hirshfield, *The Lost Reform: The Campaign for Compulsory Health Insurance in the United States from 1932 to 1943* (Cambridge: Harvard University Press 1970), 32–3.

22 L.S. Reed, *Health Insurance, The Next Step in Social Security* (New York: Harper and Brothers 1937).

23 Hirshfield, *The Lost Reform*, 44–5.

24 Ibid., 66.

25 E.E. Witte, "Organized Labor and Social Security," in M. Derber and
   E. Young, eds., *Labor and the New Deal* (Madison: University of Wisconsin Press 1957), 259.
26 E. Young, "The Split in the Labor Movement," in Derber and Young,
   eds., *Labor and the New Deal*. M. Josephson, *Sidney Hillman, Statesman
   of American Labor* (Garden City, NY: Doubleday 1952).
27 M. Derber, "Growth and Expansion," in Derber and Young, eds., *Labor and the New Deal*.
28 B. Karsh and P.L. Garman, "The Impact of the Political Left," in Derber and Young, eds., *Labor and the New Deal*.
29 Witte, "Organized Labor dans Social Security," 262.
30 Ibid., 258.
31 Hirshfield, *The Lost Reform*, chap. 5.
32 M. Harrington, *Socialism* (New York: Saturday Review Press 1972),
   263.
33 S. Perlman, *Labor in the New Deal Decade* (New York: Educational Department, International Ladies' Garment Workers' Union 1945), 32–3.
34 S.M. Lipset, *Agrarian Socialism* (Berkeley: University of California Press
   1950), 123–4.
35 T.J. Lowi, *The End of Liberalism* (New York: W.W. Norton 1969), 102–
   15.
36 Horowitz, *Canadian Labour in Politics*, 38–40 and 33. See also W.D.
   Young, *The Anatomy of a Party: The National CCF, 1932–61* (Toronto:
   University of Toronto Press 1969).
37 M.J. Brodie and J. Jenson, *Crisis, Challenge and Change: Party and Class
   In Canada* (Toronto: Methuen 1980).
38 Lipset, *Agrarian Socialism*. F.B. Roth, G.W. Meyers, F.D. Mott, and
   L.S. Rosenfield, "The Saskatchewan Experience in Payment for Hospital Care," *American Journal of Public Health* 43 (1953): 752–6. R.F.
   Badgley and S. Wolfe, *Doctors' Strike: Medical Care and Conflict in Saskatchewan* (Toronto: Macmillan of Canada 1967).
39 J. Porter, *The Vertical Mosaic* (Toronto: University of Toronto Press
   1965), 378. M.G. Taylor, *Health Insurance and Canadian Public Policy:
   The Seven Decisions That Created the Canadian Health Insurance System*
   (Montreal: McGill-Queens University Press 1978).
40 G. Hatcher, "Canadian Approaches to Health Policy Decisions – National Health Insurance," *American Journal of Public Health* 68 (1978):
   881–9. R. Roemer and M.I. Roemer, *Health Manpower Policy under National Health Insurance – The Canadian Experience* (Washington: U.S. Department of Health, Education and Welfare, DHEW Publication (HRA)
   77–37 1977). M. LeClair, "The Canadian Health Care System," in
   S. Andreopoulos, ed., *National Health Insurance: Can We Learn from
   Canada?* (New York: John Wiley and Sons 1975).

41 Taylor, *Health Insurance and Canadian Public Policy*, chap. 4. See V. Walters, "State, Capital and Labour: The Introduction of Federal-Provincial Insurance for Physician Care in Canada," *Canadian Review of Sociology and Anthropology* 19 (1982): 157–72, for a somewhat different view.

42 Lipset, *Agrarian Socialism*, 270.

43 T.R. Marmor, *The Politics of Medicare* (Chicago: Aldine Publishing Company 1973), 17.

44 Ibid.

45 S. Strickland, *Politics, Science, and Dread Disease* (Cambridge: Harvard University Press 1972).

46 J. Colombotos, "Physicians and Medicare: A Before-After Study of the Effects of Legislation on Attitudes," *American Sociological Review* 34 (1969): 318–34.

47 K. Davis, *National Health Insurance: Benefits, Costs, and Consequences* (Washington: Brookings Institute 1975), 89.

48 E.M. Kennedy, *In Critical Condition: The Crisis in American Health Care* (New York: Simon and Schuster 1972).

49 K.P. Phillips, *The Emerging Republican Majority* (New Rochelle, NY: Arlington House 1969).

50 *New York Times*, 7 Sept. 1982.

51 R. Mullner, S. Andes, R. Tatalovich, and B. Bardes, "A Spatial Analysis of Voting on Health Care Issues: United States House of Representatives, 96th Congress, First Session," *Social Science and Medicine* 16 (1982): 1147–56.

52 I.S. Falk, "Medical Care in the U.S.A.: 1932–1972: Problems, Proposals and Programs from the Committee on the Costs of Medical Care to the Committee for National Health Insurance," *Milbank Memorial Fund Quarterly* 51 (1973): 1–32. V.R. Fuchs, "From Bismarck to Woodcock: The "Irrational" Pursuit of National Health Insurance," *Journal of Law and Economics* 19 (1976): 347–59. W.P. Reuther, "The Health Care Crisis: Where Do We Go from Here?" *American Journal of Public Health* 59 (1969): 12–19.

The Canadian Health-Care System: A Developmental Overview

EUGENE VAYDA AND
RAISA B. DEBER

Canada's health-care system, although distinctive, contains elements recognizable to students of health care in the United States and the United Kingdom. At its core is a government-run insurance plan that uses public funds to pay for a private system. Medical-care services are provided primarily by physicians trained in the North American style; indeed, Canadian and American medical schools are accredited by a common body. Patients have free choice of physicians, who in turn are paid by the provincial plans on a fee-for-service basis. Public hospitals receive most of their budgets directly from government. Although national health insurance is among the most popular government programs, in recent years the declining economy and increasing health-care costs have produced pressure for cost containment similar to that which has occurred in virtually every other developed country. Since nearly three-quarters of the public expenditures for health care in Canada are for institutional and physician services, these sectors of the health-care system have come under increasing government scrutiny. The institutional sector is particularly vulnerable because it alone accounts for about half of the government-paid health-care expenditures, with an annual rate of increase above inflation.

To understand the genesis of the current system, one must first consider its constitutional matrix. Under the British North America (BNA) Act of 1867 (now known as the Constitution Act 1982), all matters of national concern, plus those activities likely to be costly, were assigned to the federal government, which had, obviously, the broadest tax base. In the health field Ottawa was given jurisdiction over quarantine, marine hospitals, and health services for native peoples and the armed forces. The provinces were given authority for those local concerns that were, all the time, thought unlikely to be costly – including roads, education, and "the Establishment, Maintenance and Management of Hospitals, Asylums, Charities, and Eleemosynary Institutions in and for the Province other than Marine Hospitals." Municipal governments have only such powers as are delegated to them by the provinces.

Health care was seen as a natural extension of hospitals and as such a provincial responsibility. Thus it must be recognized that Canada has never had a national health-care system; it has ten provincial health-care systems plus two in the northern territories (where the federal government played a more direct role). However, the escalation in health-care costs and disparities in provincial wealth soon involved the federal government in financing health services. Ottawa could therefore use fiscal levers to exert an influence on health policy despite its lack of constitutional authority; as discussed below, this has occurred repeatedly during the development of the Canadian health-insurance system.[1]

HEALTH INSURANCE IN CANADA

Although universal health insurance was first proposed in 1919, it was not enacted until much later. Local governments, industries, and voluntary agencies instead developed a variety of pre-payment plans in the 1920s and 1930s that inevitably left some services not covered and some people not insured.

Following the Depression of the 1930s and the Second World War, the federal and provincial governments turned their attention towards domestic matters. A federal-provincial conference convened in 1945 to consider programs of social reform proposed universal health insurance with federal-provincial cost-sharing. The conference also produced a draft health-care bill for the provinces, partly modelled on the United Kingdom National Health System proposal. The bill provided for patient registration with family physicians in health regions; these physicians would be responsible for their patient "lists" and paid on a capitation basis. They would also be paid additional sums to provide prevention services as medical-health officers. Services would be provided, wherever possible, in health centres. The plan would have been administered in each province under the direction of a commission representing both consumers and the professions. Although the 1945 proposals were viewed favourably by the public and key professional groups, including the

Canadian Medical Association, they failed to be enacted because they were viewed as federal incursions into provincial jurisdiction.[2]

None the less, hospital facilities were perceived to be insufficient in number, inadequate, and outdated, and government action was seen to be necessary. In lieu of a full health-insurance program, the federal government made grants for planning and hospital construction available to the provinces. This marked the first acceptance of the concept of federal-provincial cost-sharing for health services, a principle that has been the foundation of all subsequent health policy in Canada.[3]

Hospitals and hospital care in Canada had previously been financed by municipal governments, religious groups, voluntary insurance programs, and patient payments. As facilities were built and modernized with government help, this funding base became increasingly inadequate, particularly in the hospital sector. By 1955 five provinces had enacted universal hospital-insurance plans to stabilize their hospital funding. These plans, though politically popular, proved expensive. The five provinces soon pressed the federal government to honour its 1945 hospital-insurance cost-sharing offer by enacting nation-wide universal hospital insurance. Financial incentives in the ensuing Hospital Insurance and Diagnostic Services Act (HIDS) induced all provinces to adopt universal hospital insurance by 1961. Under the act, services were insured and eligible for 50 per cent federal cost-sharing only when provided in hospitals; there were no incentives to use less expensive sites. (Proposals to cover home care, for example, were not adopted.) Moreover, although universal hospital insurance in Canada provided payment to hospitals, it did not mandate an organizational framework to increase efficiency or prevent duplication of services. As a result, hospital-based patterns of practice, paid for by the provinces with "fifty-cent dollars," were solidified, leading to some of the current financial problems.

Hospital construction continued; between 1961 and 1971 the number of hospital beds in Canada increased twice as rapidly as the population (33 per cent, as compared to 18 per cent). Bed occupancy, which tends to correlate with bed availability, remained at about 80 per cent.[4] Thus, per capita utilization was also increasing. More recently, in response both to budgetary restraints and technological advances that permit greater use of out-patient care, hospitals have been pressured to reduce their bed numbers.[5]

With hospital expenditures covered, public pressure grew to insure medical-care costs. By this time, however, the concept of state-administered medical-care insurance was opposed by powerful providers, including the Canadian Medical Association and the private insurance companies. In 1961 the federal government set up a royal commission headed by a Supreme Court judge (the Hall Commission) to study health services in Canada.[6] While it was deliberating, the province of Saskatchewan enacted universal medical-care insurance. That program survived a twenty-one-day doctor's strike to become both popular and successful. In 1964 the Hall Commission delivered its lengthy report. Among its many recommendations was one that the federal government cost-share a universal medical-insurance program based on the Saskatchewan model. The resulting Medical Care Act of 1968 incorporated some of Hall's recommendations; however, it did not include his suggested reorganization of medical-services delivery. A decade later Hall was again asked to study (in less depth) the existing health-care system. As will be noted, he used the opportunity to repeat many of his previous recommendations.

The Medical Care Act, like the previous Hospital Insurance and Diagnostic Services Act, removed financial barriers but entrenched the most expensive means of delivering services; this time federal-provincial cost-sharing was allowed for those services provided by physicians. Although other health professionals may be allowed to bill the provincial insurance plans in some provinces, for the most part such services are not required under the terms of the federal program.

Because the federal government had no direct jurisdiction in health care, both the hospital and medical-care insurance programs were co-operative and voluntary. To qualify for federal-provincial cost-sharing, the provincial program had only to meet certain terms of reference:

1 Universal coverage, on uniform terms and conditions, "that does not impede, or preclude, either directly or indirectly whether by charges made to insured persons or otherwise, reasonable access to insured services by insured persons" (95 per cent of the population, without exclusion, had to be covered within two years of provincial adoption of the plan);
2 Portability of benefits from province to province;
3 Comprehensive insurance for all medically necessary services;
4 A publicly administered non-profit program.

Not only did federal-provincial cost-sharing stimulate the provinces to adopt health-insurance programs; it also served as a means of income redistribution between the wealthier and poorer provinces. The 50 per cent federal share was distributed as follows: each province was paid 25 per cent of the per capita costs it incurred for hospital in-patient services plus 25 per cent of the national average per capita cost; this sum was then multiplied by the province's population. For medical insurance, each province received 50 per cent of the average national per capita medical-care expenditure multiplied by its population. As a result, the wealthier provinces that spent more received less than 50 per cent of their costs. The differentials were especially apparent for medical-care cost-sharing, which was entirely based on national rates. In 1973–74, for example, Ontario received 49.4 per cent of its hospital costs and 44.8 per cent of its medical-care costs from federal contributions; at the other end of the spectrum, Newfoundland received 57.6 per cent of its hospital and 81.5 per cent of its medical-care costs from the federal government.[7]

It was soon evident that the federal government had no control over the total amounts expended by the provinces and received no political credit for its contributions. After initial unilateral attempts by the federal government to limit its contributions without other-wise altering the program, the federal and provincial governments settled on a new fiscal formula in 1977. Bill c-37 (Federal-Provincial Fiscal Arrangements and Established Programs Financing Act, com-monly known as EPF) reduced the direct federal contribution for health care to 25 per cent of total 1975–76 expenditures and tied any subsequent increases in federal payments to the growth of the gross national product (GNP) after 1975. To compensate, federal income and corporate taxes were decreased in order to create "tax room" for the provinces, which could (and did) increase their tax rates to balance the federal reductions without increasing total taxation levels.[8] Additional revenues required to meet any cost increases in excess of growth in the GNP would be primarily the responsibility of the provinces rather than, as in previous years, a responsibility shared with the federal government. Cost control was thereby shifted to the provinces, where both the constitutional authority for health care and the management of health-care services rest. Similar treatment was given to post-secondary education, another expensive and formerly open-ended cost-shared program under provincial jurisdiction.

EPF did not alter the four requirements for provincial health-insurance programs. However, the federal contributions for health care and post-secondary education were no longer earmarked but became part of general provincial revenues. Both health and post-secondary education now had to compete for dollars with other provincially funded programs. Some federal ability to "steer" prov-incial programs continued because the original terms of reference were retained and a series of additional per capita grants tied to specific programs were adopted (for example, grants to try to reduce the hospital focus by developing potentially less costly services like home care and extended care). None the less the overall federal capacity to steer programs was reduced. Since reporting requirements were eased, it was also difficult for the federal government to monitor compliance with its terms of reference. The federal government was thus pursuing two policies that might be seen as contradictory; it wished to alter the EPF fiscal agreements to reduce its financial commitments further, while increasing its control over health policy. In recent years limiting federal transfers have had a higher policy priority with the national government; the resulting erosion in the cash portion of federal transfers has sparked concern over whether the continuation of these trends would mean loss of any ability to enforce national standards.[9]

Among the most controversial issues was the question of direct charges to patients beyond the level paid by the provincial health-insurance plan, whether these be levied by institutions ("user charges") or physicians ("extra billing"). To many, such charges threatened to erode medicare. In 1984, after considerable discussion and despite widespread opposition from organized medicine and the provincial governments, the federal government moved to eliminate such charges through passage of the Canada Health Act (Bill C-3). This act stipulated that federal payments to the provinces would be reduced, on a dollar-for-dollar basis, by the amount of user charges by hospitals and extra billings by physicians. Direct federal prohibition was impossible because, constitutionally, health care is a provincial responsibility. However, Quebec had already in essence banned such charges, and all other provinces eliminated them before the expiration of the three-year grace period.[10] Such charges did not always go quietly; in Ontario the passage of legislation (Bill 94) to eliminate extra charges led to a month-long, unsuccessful doctor's strike. A court challenge by organized medicine to the Ontario and federal legislation also resulted, but was eventually withdrawn. By 1987 the Canada Health Act's formal goal of universal comprehensive first-dollar coverage across Canada had been met. However, as the federal cash payment has declined, provinces have again expressed an interest in user fees. For example, Quebec's recent Reform Centred on the Citizen has proposed a five-dollar user fee for "unnecessary" emergency room visits,[11] while Alberta's Rainbow Report proposed using a "smart card" with a per capita limitation on health spending.[12] The user-fee issue is evidently not yet dead.

Although EPF accentuated differences among provinces as the federal role decreased, essential similarities across the provincial plans remain. Virtually every Canadian has comprehensive medical and hospital insurance, with no co-payments permitted for insured services delivered within the province. Most hospitals are paid by provincial governments on the basis of negotiated budgets. Most physicians are paid fee-for-service on the basis of provincially negotiated fee schedules.

Taxes and premiums collected by federal and provincial governments finance the publicly funded health-care system. Although public administration was mandated from the outset of universal hospital insurance, the medical-insurance plans allowed for a brief transition period during which private health-insurance companies continued to operate. However, private health insurance now plays almost no part in the universal plan, covering only supplemental benefits (such as semi-private accommodation and other amenities) and, in some provinces, service out of country (service in other provinces is covered, in theory, under the portability arrangements). Services by other professional groups are financed in a number of ways. Hospital-based workers are usually paid through the government-funded hospital budgets. The decision about which other kinds of health practitioners can bill the provincial insurance plans varies across Canada; in some provinces, for example, chiropractors can bill directly with dollar limitations. Most usually, out-patient non-physician professional services are covered to some extent if ordered by a physician (for example, physiotherapy), while other services are excluded from the plan altogether (for example, dentistry).

Initially, most provinces administered the programs with quasi-public medical care and/or hospital commissions. In recent years most of these provincial hospital and medical-care commissions have been eliminated and their functions assumed by the provincial ministries of health. Outside of the formal health-care plans, patient self-help groups are becoming increasingly active, while other health-related activities fall under the jurisdiction of other ministries such as community services, social services, labour, or housing.

HEALTH CARE UNDER UNIVERSAL INSURANCE

In 1965 the total cost of all health-care services in Canada was $3.3 billion, in 1970 $6 billion, in 1975 more than $11 billion, and in 1985 almost $40 billion. Of the total health-care expenditures in 1985, approximately 52 per cent went to institutional care and 22 per cent to physician services. Health-care costs now make up over 30 per cent of Ontario spending, sums that must be raised by taxes or premiums. The magnitude of these expenditures and the rate of their increase (which has continued) have captured the attention of politicians.

Following the introduction of hospital insurance, health expenditures in Canada rose, both in absolute terms and as a percentage of GNP. The proportion of GNP devoted to health care rose from 5.5 per cent in 1960 to 7.3 per cent in 1971, and actual expenditures increased from $2 billion to $7 billion (250 per cent increase).[13] The introduction of medical-care insurance has had less of an effect. Between 1971 and 1976 expenditures rose again (from $7 billion to almost $12 billion), but the per cent of GNP spent on health care remained constant at about 7 per cent until the late 1970s. As a result of low economic growth, it subsequently rose to its current level near 9 per cent.[14] However, because of government insurance, public-sector funding of health care rose from 43 per cent to 75 per cent of costs; actual government spending thus increased from about $1 billion in 1960 to $5 billion in 1971, $9 billion in 1975, $13 billion in 1978–79, and over $30 billion in 1985. The size of total health-care expenditures became more visible once governments started paying almost all the bills.

In the period before universal hospital and medical-care insurance the private sector had covered some hospital and physician care. At present over 90 per cent of the cost of hospital and physician services are paid by the public sector. Private payments are now limited primarily to nursing homes (40 per cent of costs), dental care (90 per cent) and drugs and prostheses (75 per cent).[15]

Hospital use and its attendant costs were particularly vulnerable to examination in Canada because, compared to many countries, particularly to the United States, Canada had high bed-to-population and bed-use-to-population ratios. For example, in Ontario 8.9 per cent of the population aged sixty-five and over were in an institution on any one day, a higher utilization rate than in the United States or the United Kingdom.[16] While a small portion of the higher Canadian bed use could be explained by its remote and isolated north, which was served by many small hospitals, some was a reflection of increased bed supply. By 1971 Canada had 23 per cent more hospital beds per capita than the United States and used 30 per cent more hospital days per capita.[17]

FEDERAL AND PROVINCIAL PLANNING REPORTS

Beginning in the late 1960s, concern regarding the above-inflation increases in health-care expenditures was reflected in a number of government planning reports that identified rising expenditures and stressed the need for greater efficiency and the provision of less-expensive forms of health-service delivery. Their goal was not necessarily to cut costs but rather to contain the rate of increase. They were influenced by a strong body of expert opinion calling for improving the efficiency and containing the costs of the health-care system through such measures as shifting from in-patient to out-patient care, reducing the number of hospital beds, and promoting paramedical workers and community-health (and social-service) centres. This emphasis was further justified by the work of Illich, Fuchs, and McKeown, which challenged both the efficacy and the marginal benefits of further increases in health-care expenditures in developed countries.[18] At the national level a 1969 task force on the costs of health services concluded that increased costs could only be dealt with by reduced standards of care, increased taxes, premiums and/or deterrent fees, or more efficient operation of the system.[19] The 1973 report of the Community Health Centre Project, commonly known as the Hastings Report,[20] recommended the large-scale development of community health centres by the provinces as well as reorganization and integration of all health services and reduction in the number of hospital beds. The Lalonde Report of the federal Department of National Health and Welfare, in what some have termed primarily a government justification for reduced spending for personal health-care services, stressed the importance of health promotion, lifestyle modification, and greater individual responsibility for health instead of increased provision of medical services.[21]

Many provincial governments conducted or commissioned their own studies, all of which reached similar conclusions. The 1972 Manitoba white paper on health suggested regionalization of health services and the establishment of community-health and social-services centres in order to shift from hospital to ambulatory-care services.[22] In Quebec a 1970 four-volume health section of the report of the Commission of Inquiry on Health and Social Welfare, known as the Castonguay Report, also suggested decentralization, community clinics, and greater consumer input into the organization of health-care services.[23] A 1973 report commissioned by the recently elected New Democratic party government of British Columbia recommended complete reorganization of the British Columbia health-care system with regionalization and rationalization based on Community Health Resource and Health Centres and a de-emphasis on hospital use.[24] In Ontario the 1970 report of the Committee on the Healing Arts, the 1976 Health Report of the Ontario Economic

Council, and the 1974 report of the Health Planning Task Force, known as the Mustard Report, all identified increased cost, excessive use of hospital services and the control and deployment of medical and health manpower as key issues, and included rationalization, regionalization, and deinstitutionalization among their remedies.[25]

Although most of these recommendations were never implemented, the concepts contained within the reports are now being more actively debated and have given rise to a new slew of provincial reports.[26] This largely ideological debate about the roles and responsibilities of physicians, other providers, government, and the public has been forced on the system because of the worsening economic climate in Canada and the perceived need to control cost escalation in health care and other publicly funded programs.

THE HALL REVIEW OF HEALTH SERVICES

Canadian health insurance was a mix of public funding and private practice. The universal system initially paid the bills but did not attempt to manage the programs. Providers, particularly physicians, were (and still are) treated as private entrepreneurs who happen to operate in a publicly funded system. Hospitals have continued under community control with independent boards of trustees. However, virtually all of their budgets are now determined and paid by provincial governments; some cost-containment in the hospital sector has thus been possible, although changes in hospital governance had not yet become an issue.

During the 1970s the percentage of GNP spent on health care remained constant at about 7 per cent. Although health economists hailed this as an example of successful containment, providers (both physicians and hospitals) charged that the system was underfunded, and demanded that more money be devoted to health care. If public funds were not available, physicians and hospital administrators favoured the injection of private money through user charges and private insurance. Opting out and extra billing by physicians increased, and negotiations between provincial governments and their doctors became more acrimonious. Confrontations resulted, and in many provinces work stoppages and rotating strikes took place. Hospital budgets that had been calculated on a line-by-line basis were converted in most provinces to global budgets, and the annual rates of increase were frequently less than the rate of inflation. Hospitals protested these "inadequate" increases both privately and publicly and were not infrequently successful in obtaining additional money to cover their budgetary deficits.

It was in the context of confrontation and charges of underfunding of the health-care system that the federal government in 1979 asked Justice Emmet Hall to examine the universal health-insurance program his 1964 royal commission report had recommended. Specifically, he was asked to examine two charges: that the total federal contribution plus the "tax room" was resulting in fewer health-care dollars for the provinces; and that, since these monies were no longer earmarked for health care, the provinces were diverting them to other programs. He was also asked to examine extra billing and the adversarial relationship that had developed between provincial governments and their physicians.

Hall concluded that both of the charges were false: the federal contributions plus "tax room" were actually producing more money than the earlier cost-sharing formula would have, and the provinces were not diverting these dollars from health care. Both federal and provincial health-care spending was actually increasing.[27]

In his review of extra billing, Hall concluded that physicians should not be allowed to opt out or extra bill. Instead he recommended that they should be "adequately paid" and that differences between provincial governments and physicians should be settled by compulsory binding arbitration. His recommendations regarding physicians were weakened because Hall did not suggest a mechanism for determining "adequate" compensation, and provincial governments have been unwilling to accept the constraints on their spending authority implied by compliance with arbitration reports. In 1981 a federal parliamentary task force was set up on federal-provincial fiscal arrangements; it took an even stronger stand against user charges and opting out than Hall had done.[28] Although the subsequent elimination of extra billing following passage of the Canada Health Act was accompanied in some provinces with commitments to a system of binding arbitration, most provincial governments have proved unwilling to accept judgments that run contrary to their own priorities. As a result, relationships between physicians and government remain strained.[29]

CURRENT PROBLEMS

Not surprisingly, the universal health plan has encountered both difficulty and conflict. Government began by paying bills. With rising costs, government paymasters took on an increased role. They chose to use the blunt instrument of cost-containment rather than the more difficult step of modifying the organization and management of the system. As a result, providers now complain that the system is underfunded, while governments see only what they perceive as the insatiable financial appetite of the health-care system. Both charge that the system is in crisis.

When charges of crisis are carefully examined, they have proved to be unfounded. However, there are justifiable concerns that the system is rigid and inflexible and may soon be faced with a rapid increase in costs. Preservation of the autonomy of local institutions has been valued, but there has been a resulting weakness in control over the acquisition of new technology, and fears that the system is inefficient. As a result, concerns are increasingly voiced that a focus on technology coupled with an oversupply of physicians and services may have produced a system that will be unable to adapt to the problems of an aging population, a post-industrial society, and changing human-service needs. One consequence was a reorganization of the Ontario Ministry of Health, including the introduction of program management, in an attempt to focus more on health outcomes in making allocation decisions. There has also been a new flurry of planning reports from provincial governments, including the Rochon Commission in Quebec and Ontario's triumverate of Spassoff, Evans, and Podborski; these have been reviewed by Angus and Mhatre and Deber.[30] The perception that Canada's health system may be heading for trouble appears to be widespread, and cries for reform are becoming louder.

A second problem arises from Canada's current constitutional ferment. Health care, as a national program within provincial jurisdiction, may therefore be affected by efforts to restructure the federal system.[31]

A third problem arises from a trend we term "deprivatization" – the systematic tendency of government services to expand into new areas that formerly were considered private concerns. For example, there has been pressure for government to increase provision of services in areas not included under medicare, such as long-term care, assistive devices, dentistry, and even housing and provision of homemaking services.[32] The burden on government has thus continued to grow, and health expenditures to increase at well above the rate of inflation.

The federal government wishes to reduce its contributions for health care, placing more financial responsibility on the provinces. Providers are demanding more money, which they will accept from provincial governments or from the private sector. Supplemental private insurance for insured benefits continues to be prohibited. When coupled with growing provincial deficits, the provincial publicly funded health-care programmes are moving towards potentially untenable financial positions.

At least two scenarios are possible. One would place the health sector under greater government control; the government would then take a major role in the management of the system, the control of resources, and the employment of physicians. The second scenario would shift responsibility for health care away from government into the private sector. The first scenario, greater government control, implies increasing confrontation with providers and the need for tough and consistent stances by the provinces. It is also more likely to maintain the integrity of the publicly funded universal system.

The second scenario, shifting control, may be superficially more attractive. It implies a diminished provincial role (and budgetary responsibility) as private funding increases. However, this policy will lead to greater total costs for health care and possibly to a two-class hospital and medical-care system. It would also be in violation of the Canada Health Act – which requires government to fund all medically necessary services – and would be enormously unpopular with the public. Accordingly, most provincial governments appear to be moving towards greater attempts to control the system, including the threat of controls over the number of physicians allowed to bill the health-care system.

The issues are basically ideological, and after twenty-two years they can no longer be avoided, particularly when poor economic performance is coupled with a rising proportion of GNP devoted to health care.[33] The alternatives have been defined at one extreme by the system in the United Kingdom. There, costs were controlled, but physicians were essentially government employees, paid by salary or capitation rather than on a fee-for-service basis, and groups of hospitals were directed by regional authorities rather than community boards. At the other extreme is the more costly, essentially free-enterprise system in the United States, with means testing, accessibility limited by patients' finances, and government funding only for the needy.

Until now Canada has used public funds to pay for a private system. It has avoided key issues of reorganization and management of the system as a whole. Australia, in confronting similar issues, moved temporarily to a more private system,[34] but the popularity of Canada's present universal system – particularly in contrast to the American model – makes a private solution less likely here. The Canadian solution to most problems has typically been moderation and compromise. Extreme moves in either direction would thus represent an unlikely break with tradition. Contemplating those alternatives, however, will be healthy if it helps to produce the changes necessary to ensure the survival of Canada's medicare program.

NOTES

1 R.G. Evans, "'We'll Take Care of It for you': Health Care in the Canadian Community," *Daedalus* 117 (1988): 155–89; R.B. Deber, "Philosophical Underpinnings of Canada's Health Care System," *Canada u.s. Outlook* 2 (1991): 20–45; R. Van Loon and M.S. Whittington, *The Canadian Political System: Environment, Structure and Process*, 4th ed. (Toronto: McGraw-Hill Ryerson 1987).

2 M. Taylor, *Health Insurance and Canadian Public Policy*, 2nd ed. (Montreal: McGill-Queen's University Press 1987).

3 Ibid.

4 E. Vayda, R.G. Evans, and W. Mindell, "Universal Health Insurance in Canada: History, Problems, Trends," *Journal of Community Health* 4 (1979): 217–31.

5 P. Gamble, "Hospital Ressources in Metropolitan Toronto: The Reality versus the Myth," in R.B. Deber and G.G. Thompson, *Restructuring Canada's Health Services System: How Do We Get There from Here?* (Toronto: University of Toronto Press 1992).

6 Canada, *Royal Commission on Health Services* (Hall Report), summary, vol. 1 and 2 (Ottawa: Queen's Printer 1964, 1965).

7 S. Andreopoulos, ed., *National Health Insurance: Can We Learn from Canada?* (Toronto: Wiley 1975).

8 L. Soderstrom, *The Canadian Health Care System* (London: Croon Helm 1978); R.J. Van Loon, "From Shared Cost to Block Funding and Beyond: The Politics of Health Insurance in Canada," *Journal of Health Politics, Policy & Law* 2 (1978): 454–78.

9 A. Thompson, *Federal Support for Health Care* (Ottawa: HEAL, the Health Action Lobby 1991).

10 S. Heiber and R. Deber, "Banning Extra Billing in Canada: Just What the Doctor Didn't Order," *Canadian Public Policy* 13, no. 1 (Mar. 1987): 62–74; and "Freedom, Equality, and the Charter of Rights: Regulating Physician Reimbursement," *Canadian Public Administration* 31, no. 4 (Winter 1988): 566–89.

11 Quebec, *A Reform Centred On The Citizen* (Quebec: Ministère de la Santé et des Services sociaux 1989).

12 L. Hyndman, chair, *The Rainbow Report: Our Vision For Health*, Premier's Commission on Future Health Care for Albertans, 3 vols. (Edmonton 1989).

13 M.L. Barer and R.G. Evans, "Riding North on a South-bound Horse? Expenditures, Prices, Utilization and Income in the Canadian Health Care System," in R.G. Evans and G.L. Stoddart, *Medicare at Maturity* (Calgary: University of Calgary Press 1984), 53–73; R.G. Evans, "Health Care in Canada: Patterns in Funding and Regulation," in G.

McLachlan and A. Maynard, *The Public/Private Mix for Health* (London: Nuffield Provincial Hospitals Trust 1982); G.H. Hatcher, *Universal Free Health Care in Canada, 1947–1977*, NIH pub. no. 81–2052 (Washington: US Department of Health and Human Services 1981).

14 G.J. Schieber and J.-P. Poullier, "International Health Care Expenditure Trends: 1987," *Health Affairs* 8, no. 3 (Fall 1989): 169–77.

15 Barer and Evans, "Riding North."

16 M.J. Gross and C. Schwenger, *Health Care Costs for the Elderly in Ontario: 1976–2026*. (Toronto: Ontario Economic Council 1981).

17 Vayda, Evans, and Mindell, "Universal Health Insurance."

18 I. Illich, *Limits to Medicine: Medical Nemesis, The Expropriation of Health* (Toronto: McClelland & Stewart 1975); V.R. Fuchs, *Who Shall Live: Health, Economics and Social Policy* (New York: Basic Books 1974); T. McKeown, *The Role of Medicine* (Oxford: Blackwell 1979).

19 Canada, *Task Force Reports on the Cost of Health Services in Canada*, 3 vol. (Ottawa: Queen's Printer 1969).

20 J.E.F. Hastings, chair, *The Community Health Centre in Canada*, vol. 1 (Ottawa: Information Canada 1973).

21 M. Lalonde, *A New Perspective on the Health of Canadians* (Ottawa: Information Canada 1974); R. Evans, "A Retrospective on the 'New Perspective,'" *Journal of Health Politics, Policy & Law* 7 (1982): 325–44; E. Vayda, "Preventive Programs and the Political Process," *Modern Medicine in Canada* 32 (1977): 260–4.

22 Manitoba, *White Paper on Health Policy* (Winnipeg: Department of Health and Social Development 1972).

23 Quebec, *Report of the Commission of Inquiry on Health and Social Service*, part 2, tome 2, *The Health Plan* (Castonguay Report) (Quebec 1970).

24 R. Foulkes, *Health Security for British Columbians*, vol. 1 (Vancouver: Province of British Columbia 1973).

25 Ontario, *Report of the Committee on the Healing Arts*, vol. 1 (Toronto: Queen's Printer 1970); Ontario Economic Council, *Issues and Alternatives 1976: Health* (Toronto: Ontario Economic Council 1976); Ontario, *Report on the Health Planning Task Force* (Mustard Report) (Toronto: Ontario Ministry of Health 1974).

26 R.B. Deber and E. Vayda, "The Environment of Health Policy Implementation: The Ontario, Canada Example," in George Knox, ed., *Investigative Methods in Public Health*, vol. 3 of *Oxford Textbook of Public Health*, ed. Walter Holland (Oxford: Oxford University Press 1985); D.E. Angus, *Review of Significant Health Care Commissions and Task Forces in Canada since 1983–84* (Ottawa: Canadian Hospital Association Press 1991).

27 E.M. Hall, *Canada's National-Provincial Health Program of the 1980s*, Health Services Review 1979 (Saskatoon: Craft Litho 1980).

28 Canada, *Fiscal Federalism in Canada,* Report of the Parliamentary Task Force on Federal-Provincial Arrangements (Ottawa: Minister of Supply and Services 1981).

29 C.J. Tuohy, "Medicine and the State in Canada: The Extra-Billing Issue in Perspective," *Canadian Journal of Political Science* 21, no. 2 (June 1988): 267–96.

30 Angus, *Review of Significant Commissions and Task Forces,* and S.L. Mhatre and R. Deber, "From Equal Access to Health Care to Equitable Access to Health: Review of Canadian Provincial Health Commissions and Reports," *International Journal of Health Services,* forthcoming.

31 R.B. Deber, "Regulatory and Administrative Options for Canada's Health Care System," background paper prepared for HEAL, the Health Action Lobby, 8 Oct. 1991.

32 B.J. Fried, R.B. Deber and P. Leatt, "Corporatization and Deprivatization of Health Services in Canada," *International Journal of Health Services* 17, no. 4 (1987): 567–83, repr. in J. Warren Salmon, ed., *The Corporate Transformation of Health Care* (Amityville, NY: Baywood Publishing 1990), 167–86.

33 A.J. Culyer, *Health Expenditures in Canada: Myth and Reality, Past and Future* (Toronto: Canadian Tax Foundation 1988); R.G. Evans, J. Lomas, M.L. Barer, et al., "Controlling Health Expenditures – The Canadian Reality," *New England Journal of Medicine* 320, no. 9 (1989): 571–7.

34 J.S. Deeble, "Unscrambling the Omelet: Public and Private Health Care Financing in Australia," in McLachlan and Maynard, *The Public/Private Mix for Health.*

Making Canada Safe for Sex: Government and the Problem of Sexually Transmitted Disease in the Twentieth Century

JAY CASSEL

Since the First World War Canadian governments at all levels have been extensively involved in efforts to cope with sexually transmitted disease (STD). Between 1918 and 1920 most provinces passed special legislation to control STD, with Prince Edward Island following suit in 1929. Their action was prompted by the high prevalence of venereal infection in both the general public and the armed forces before and during the Great War, and it rested on the recognition of a need for special legal powers and major resources of manpower, material, and money.[1] The statutes went through some revision, chiefly between 1936 and 1947, but remained essentially unchanged until the 1970s and 1980s, when most provinces reworked their legislation into single, all-encompassing public-health acts.

Throughout the twentieth century Canadian STD programs comprised five elements: medical measures (free diagnosis and treatment); "social work" (ensuring that patients completed treatment, and identifying others who were infected); regulation of conduct (implementation of laws and regulations aimed at reducing the spread of STD); epidemiological work (accumulation of statistics to trace patterns of infection and assess progress in controlling the epidemic); and education. Heaviest emphasis was placed on medical measures. The primary goal was the elimination of the diseases from the community, much like the successful actions to eliminate smallpox, typhus, and tuberculosis. The object, in brief, was to make Canada safe for sex – a task that turned out to be very difficult.

Discussions of sexually transmitted disease have long acknowledged the significance of social influences.[2] Recent writers, following Michel Foucault and other post-structuralist thinkers, have focused on the social character of medical knowledge and practice, and the cultural definitions of normality and illness.[3] In his survey of American efforts Alan Brandt argues that venereal disease came to serve social purposes, chiefly the control of sexuality and individual conduct, and "in its transformation from a biological entity to a social symbol, venereal disease has defied control ... So long as these social *uses* of the diseases have dominated medical and public approaches, therapeutic approaches to the problem have necessarily remained secondary" – and this has impeded efforts to decrease the prevalence of the diseases in the community.[4] But the record of efforts to cope with STD in Canada would suggest that this analysis needs some revision. In focusing on particular social purposes, these authors down-play or overlook other factors that make STD such an intractable problem.

With sexually transmitted disease, there are substantial challenges of several kinds, each compounding the effects of the others. These include the biology of the organisms and the disorders they cause, medical capabilities, individual desires, and the response to disease of both those who are infected and those who are not. Sexually transmitted diseases are biological phenomena, but the condition of having an infection is bound up in social constructions. Disease does not simply exist; its existence is interpreted: people read meanings into illness. The interpretation placed by the community on the fact of having a disease will influence both the measures adopted and the actions of individuals. Legal considerations, particularly the rights and freedoms allowed or denied individuals and groups will affect public-health strategies. The resources that a community can mobilize at any particular time will also influence the scope of operations. Finally, there are administrative difficulties arising from the complex medical and social tasks involved in dealing with STD, and the friction that almost inevitably develops within systems. STD is such a difficult problem because medical difficulties coincide with social impediments and their effects are exacerbated by logistical and administrative problems.

1. SEXUALLY TRANSMITTED DISEASES

1.1 Biological Phenomena

There are at least twenty-six sexually transmitted diseases, all of which present significant challenges.[5] Six are particularly noteworthy: syphilis, gonorrhea, non-specific urethritis (NSU), chlamydia (often the cause of NSU), herpes, and the acquired immunodeficiency syndrome (AIDS). Recognizing the diseases is not easy because they often resemble other diseases – a particular problem with syphilis. In women, gonorrhea, NSU, and chlamydia may cause no obvious signs and symptoms until the infection is well advanced. Some men remain asymptomatic for a long time, while in others signs may be hidden – inside the anus, for example, a common site among homosexuals. Such periods of infectivousness without frank indications facilitate the spread of STDs. Herpes, in contrast, leads to recurrent outbreaks of painful blisters; however, early in these eruptions the disease is highly infectious but may not be painful enough to prompt preventive measures. In AIDS the immune system is debilitated and for a long time there are no frank signs or symptoms. What ultimately appears to be ailing the patient are disorders caused by "opportunistic" infections. Syphilis, gonorrhea, NSU, and chlamydia can leave a patient sterile. If a woman is infected during pregnancy, the offspring may also suffer: gonorrhea can cause blindness, while syphilis can lead to spontaneous abortions, still-births, or severe deformities. A minority of patients who get syphilis may eventually suffer serious damage to the brain, nervous system, and heart. AIDS and its attendant infections are generally fatal.

1.2 Responses to STD

Reactions to any disease have both personal and social aspects.[6] With STD, emotions are bound to be mobilized by the very fact of sexual transmission and by the alarming consequences – debility, disfigurement, sterility, blindness, insanity, death. Individual and collective responses to STD have therefore been heavily influenced by fear. From the 1940s through the 1970s the decisive treatment afforded by antibiotics greatly reduced the fears of many Canadians. Attitudes changed in the later 1970s when herpes spread rapidly and antibiotic-resistant strains of gonorrhea appeared. Although herpes was not life-threatening, there was no cure. This undermined a general sense of security in the powers of medicine. The fear or paranoia that accompanied the rise of AIDS in the 1980s was thus not new. Nor is it surprising that public concern should be so strong: AIDS has a horrifying finality exceeding the threat of earlier maladies, and there is no definitive treatment.

Closely related to this response is the fear of contagion. This arose from the collective memory in Western societies of great epidemics such as polio in the 1940s and 1950s, influenza, especially in 1918–

19, and recurring outbreaks of smallpox, diphtheria, scarlet fever, and cholera in the nineteenth century. Popular conceptions of the organisms associated with STD were distorted by common, highly contagious viral diseases like the flu and the common cold. When AIDS appeared and was found to be caused by a virus, many assumed that the organism could have similar capabilities.

Perceptions of STD are also mirrored in the metaphors used in discussing measures.[7] Military activity had a particularly strong appeal, contributing words such as "campaign," "strategy," "combat," "attack," and "eradicate." The primary element in this metaphor was "enemy" – in this instance, an organism. "Carriers," those with the enemy already lurking unseen inside them, would become associated with the enemy and therefore themselves became targets. Such language contributed to perceptions of the "otherness" of those with a disease, setting them up as alien to the general populace.

In the absence of a satisfactory empirical or mechanistic explanation, disease has often been interpreted as a personal failing, perhaps constitutional but usually in some way moral. Some aspect of the individual's conduct violated the social order, which was believed to coincide with the natural order, and that violation led to a natural catastrophe, physical illness. Individuals thus became responsible for their illness, "acquiring" disease by virtue of their lifestyle, diet, or psychological nature. Disease, then, became a way to oblige others to adhere to a form of conduct that people assumed would make social existence more satisfactory for everyone in a community. The classic example of disease being given a moral construction is, of course, STD.

Public discussion of STD in Canada during much of the period under study was closely linked to the prevailing interpretation of human sexuality.[8] The patriarchal social system prevalent in the Western world created a "double standard" about sexual conduct. During the first half of the twentieth century many believed that the human male had a strong "sex drive" and was quite likely to respond to it. This led, on the one hand, to determined efforts to curb men's sexual urges and, on the other, to a certain acceptance of male sexual activity beyond the confines of married life. It followed that men might have sex with several women, especially before they married. By contrast, women were thought to have more subdued sexual urges, and would therefore limit the expression of their sexuality to a single mate in a marital setting. Women were divided into "ladies" who adhered to this cultural ideal and "loose women" who did not.

The predominant epidemiological model for sexually transmitted diseases during the first half of the period under study actually incorporated these assumptions. Because the human male had a strong "sex drive," he might have sex with several women and would therefore run the risk of getting an infection. The position of women in the model was quite different. At first it was thought that only prostitutes and "loose women" were involved. These few women had many male partners. The men, though more numerous, had fewer contacts individually. In the minds of the men who dominated the medical establishment it seemed to follow that a few women were responsible for spreading much of the disease. The full logic of this view was never pressed. It would have been entirely consistent to argue that there were actually many male carriers and relatively few female carriers. Instead, articles, pamphlets, and lectures concentrated on the role of prostitutes and "loose women" in spreading disease and on the fact that men would "fall prey" to them. Women who decided to have sex out of wedlock and with different men were condemned with vigour. Authorities considered this distinctly "hazardous" behaviour. It was also most at variance with what the moral code dictated as acceptable female behaviour.

During the Second World War research revealed that very few women who had sex with members of the Canadian armed forces were paid prostitutes; "pick-ups" accounted for over 90 per cent of contacts.[9] Several times between the 1940s and 1970s the epidemiological model was revised to account for the greater numbers of women evidently involved. Ideas were most dramatically revised during the "sexual revolution" of the 1960s. But it was a long time before public-health activists saw the need to address not just the male "sex drive" but women's desires as well.

Ideas about the pattern of transmission led people to take STD as a sign of certain kinds of sexual activity. The diseases were long perceived as largely a problem of certain groups, such as prostitutes, "bohemians," and drug addicts. The reaction of many people to a problem such as STD, one that was already in the community but had not yet affected them directly, was to distance themselves from those involved and then to condemn whatever made the other people different. Indeed, the higher prevalence of disease among these marginalized groups served to drive them further to the limits of acceptability. STD could be interpreted as evidence of social decay and a departure from Judaeo-Christian views of the sanctity and permanence of heterosexual marriage and family life. The diseases therefore prompted another kind of fear, one focused on the social order.

With a certain concept of the pattern of transmission also came a view of who was responsible.[10] In Judeo-Christian thought, disease has often been interpreted as a mark of God's displeasure or punishment for misconduct. In Western culture the theme recurs: people *choose* to behave in ways that lead to infection; STD was seen as a voluntarily acquired malady. People with an STD were stereotyped as promiscuous, hedonistic, self-indulgent. With this perception came the common notion that disease in some way provided rough justice: "guilt" brought "punishment" – social ostracism, restricted liberty, financial burdens.

Fear of certain forms of sexuality also underlies responses to STD. This has been particularly evident with homosexuality, which jeopardized many Canadians' sense of their own sexual identity and the social order.[11] Homosexuality was a criminal offence in Canada until 1969, and legislation against same-sex activity was periodically tightened between the 1880s and the 1950s. During the twentieth century public awareness of homosexuality slowly increased, especially with the publication of the Kinsey reports on male (1948) and female (1953) sexual behaviour in the United States. The 1950s were actually a period of intensified efforts to limit homosexual activity in Canada, as in the United States and the United Kingdom. While Canadians began to widen the bounds of what was good or acceptable sexual behaviour, they sought to offset the new conditions by more rigidly defining what was unacceptable, including nearly all forms of homosexual activity. But an increasing number of people found even the broadened definitions unsatisfactory, and a process of criticism and revolt led to further changes in the 1960s. In 1969 clauses in the Canadian Criminal Code making homosexual acts illegal were largely but not entirely eliminated. An increasingly free expression of gay and lesbian sexuality ensued, although the struggle for acceptance continued.

During the second half of the twentieth century, revelations that STD was common among homosexuals intensified the popular sense of how "wrong" this form of sexuality was. Those who condemned homosexuality could persuade themselves that while an organism might cause the disease, it was a lifestyle that turned it into a public catastrophe. The label "risk group," often employed in epidemiological discussions, contributed to the sense of a "tainted community" separate from the self-styled moral and healthy majority. When it appeared, AIDS affected gays and intravenous drug users in particular, two groups that were already marginalized and therefore vulnerable to attack. In Canada as elsewhere, some people wanted to segregate those with AIDS, oust them from jobs, or prevent them from living in their midst.[12]

2. THE MAGNITUDE OF THE PROBLEM

Given the nature of STD, it is hardly surprising that complete and reliable data have always been hard to obtain. Shortly before the First World War physicians concluded that between 5 and 15 per cent of all Canadians had syphilis and several times as many had had gonorrhea at some time in their lives. These figures were based on extrapolation from disease patterns among people seeking medical care, and doubtless represent an overestimate. All the signs, however, indicate that STD was remarkably widespread.[13]

During the First World War Canadians found that their army had the highest incidence of venereal infection in Western Europe.[14] By the end of the war there were 66,083 cases, 15.8 per cent of the Canadian Expeditionary Force. Repeat infections and relapses make it unlikely that the number of men infected was quite that high. None the less, the huge caseload was directly responsible for the government's decision to organize diagnosis, treatment, and education measures for the armed forces and then for the civilian population.

Between the two world wars reporting was erratic and incomplete. It appears that minor STDs declined markedly, and severe complications of syphilis, gonorrhea, and NSU were less common. However, the number of new cases of the principal diseases hardly changed.[15]

During the Second World War the incidence of STDs again rose. In 1940 6.2 per cent of all men in the army developed a venereal infection, though only 3 per cent of those overseas did. In 1943–4 figures stood at 3 per cent of soldiers in Canada, compared with 3.4 per cent of those overseas. In 1945, especially after the advent of peace in Europe, figures shot up – despite the introduction of penicillin. In Canada 3.7 per cent were infected, while overseas the figure for the year as a whole stood at 6.8 per cent.[16] In the civilian population the incidence of syphilis and gonorrhea had been rising since 1937, though the number of unreported cases remained uncertain. In 1945, 15,279 cases of syphilis were reported, the highest number to date. The rate of venereal infection, based on reported cases alone, increased more than threefold. The overall figures for 1945 (336 per 100,000) and 1946 (338.3) were the highest in the twentieth century.[17]

Wartime VD campaigns may have prompted more reporting. More important, however, was the social upheaval that loosened former restraints. Observers noted that increased activity extended to younger people, including teenagers.[18] Not surprisingly, the medical breakthrough of penicillin did not bring about any major or immediate changes in the prevalence of STD. Then again, there were problems with sulpha drugs, and penicillin was in short supply.

Between 1948 and 1960 statistics were more encouraging. By the early 1950s the rates of infection for the principal diseases, syphilis and gonorrhea, had fallen to one-third of the wartime high. In the mid-1950s, however, the favourable trends slowed, then reversed. [19]

From the 1960s to the 1980s the incidence and prevalence of sexually transmitted diseases in Canada rose again – much as they did across the Western world. [20] At first figures increased slowly, then shot up at the end of the 1960s, continuing to increase sharply through the 1970s and early 1980s, by which time they were two to two and one-half times higher than in the 1950s. The chief concerns were gonorrhea and NSU. By contrast, syphilis did not rise much; cases increased appreciably between 1972 and 1977 but declined again in the 1980s. In 1981 gonorrhea reached an all-time peak of 56,336 cases, which surpassed the record rate for the disease set in 1945–46. Officials estimated that the actual amount was between two and three times the number reported. Regulations did not require reporting of other diseases; however, laboratory reports of chlamydial infection increased fivefold in the first half of the 1980s, the great majority of cases being female and an ever-increasing number in the fifteen- to nineteen-year age bracket. A major increase in ectopic pregnancies was believed to be due in some measure to fallopian-tube damage from STD, chiefly gonorrhea and chlamydia. Alongside these problems, the incidence of genital herpes rapidly accelerated in the later 1970s. This prompted governments to add it to the list of reportable diseases. In 1986, 14,000 cases were reported, but officials estimated that the real number was 20,000 to 50,000 cases a year.

Why did the incidence of STD begin to rise again? During the 1960s and early 1970s it was common to blame the change on "the three Ps": permissiveness, promiscuity, and the pill. But the downward trends in the incidence of STD had stopped by the second half of the 1950s, well before the "sexual revolution." Condoms, the principal contraceptive device in Canada until the mid-1960s, had provided a barrier that reduced chances of infection; oral contraceptives and intra-uterine devices (IUDs) did not. In some circles changing attitudes favoured increased sexual activity: pre-marital sex, multiple partners, sexual activity by those in their teens, and oral or anal sexual practices became more common. Demographics undoubtedly played a significant role as well. During the 1950s and early 1960s there was a great increase in the number of people in their teens and twenties, age groups traditionally among the most active sexually. The population was increasingly urban, and with concentration of population came greater opportunities for multiple contacts. Disease patterns were probably also affected by mass transit, the car culture, and easier travel to points around the globe. The rise in caseloads also reflects improved detection: in the 1970s gonorrhea and NSU were sought more diligently by primary-care physicians, and better techniques to detect diseases were developed.

One group whose figures were distinct from the general patterns was male homosexuals.[21] Discussion of homosexuality, and the association of homosexual activities with STD, did not appear in Canadian medical journals until the early 1950s – after Kinsey's report on male sexuality. Indeed, for the first half of the twentieth century STD was perceived primarily as a heterosexual problem, very much in contrast to later perceptions. Canadian physicians subsequently recognized that levels of STD were much higher in the homosexual community than in the general population. For example, in the 1970s a very high proportion of syphilis cases (as much as half) were found to be homosexual or bisexual men. Hepatitis B, a potentially serious liver infection, was also several times more common among homosexual than among heterosexual men.

Observers attributed the patterns to several factors. One feature of gay liberation from the late 1960s on into the early 1980s was a belief that sexual activity need not be limited in any way. The combination of multiple partners, sometimes a great many, drawn from a relatively small group, increased the chances of exposure to disease, as did the difficulty of seeing or otherwise detecting some infections. Conditions were exacerbated by legal sanctions and the hostile attitudes of the public, including a significant number of physicians.

The acquired immunodeficiency syndrome (AIDS) was recognized in the second half of 1981 and first appeared among homosexual men. In Canada cases continued to be predominantly gay men aged twenty to fifty, despite some extension to the heterosexual community, initially through infected blood products and contaminated needles and latterly through sexual transmission. The number of new cases in Canada increased at an alarming rate, from 22 in 1982 to 1,017 in 1989. By the end of the decade the total was just over 3,200; 58 per cent were already dead.[22] Over 16,000 Canadians were known to be seropositive, and some epidemiologists estimated that the true total was between 30,000 and 50,000.

3. DIRECTION AND FUNDING

To understand the performance of Canadian STD programs, it is useful to begin by considering the nature of their direction and financial support.

3.1 *Direction*

Under the vague terms of the British North America Act, public health, and with it STD control, appeared to be primarily a provincial responsibility. In the aftermath of the First World War the provinces established VD divisions within their boards or departments of health. These divisions were to provide medical services, receive and follow reports of all cases, and direct a public-education program. Municipal governments were to operate local-treatment clinics with financial assistance from the province. The provinces also undertook to perform tests for patients of private physicians and to supply drugs for them at no charge.

The BNA Act notwithstanding, federal involvement began in 1919, when the Department of Health was first created. Its special Division of Venereal Disease Control had the second largest budget in the department, most of it to be distributed to provincial programs. The idea was that the federal VD division would serve as a co-ordinating centre for health work and would assist provincial programs financially, ensuring that basic measures were uniformly operating across the country. To receive funds, the provinces had to meet certain conditions: diagnosis and treatment had to be provided free of charge at special clinics and hospitals; anyone in custody who had VD was to be treated; diagnosis laboratories were to be operated; and a provincial VD division had to be maintained that would supervise all operations, including an education campaign. These arrangements persisted until the federal grant was ended in 1931. The VD Division itself ceased to exist in 1934, a victim of Depression-era restraint. When war broke out in 1939, public-health activists pressed for renewed action, but the federal government was slow to respond. Finally, in 1943 the VD Division was re-established, and this arrangement lasted from the 1940s to the 1960s. [23]

Public sex education was controversial, and government action was full of compromises. [24] While education programs have been maintained in a fitful way ever since 1919, the federal and provincial governments usually undertook only limited programs of their own, preferring to entrust much of the actual work to private organizations particularly concerned with health and education. Government efforts were largely directed at the production of posters and pamphlets. The most important private organization in the 1920s and 1930s was the Canadian National Council for Combating Venereal Disease, soon renamed the Canadian Social Hygiene Council, and later the Health League of Canada. It relied heavily on government grants, becoming in effect the officially approved medium of STD education. But by maintaining a separate, private organization, governments were able to insulate themselves from any controversy that might arise. Indeed, the federal government withdrew from all work by the mid-1920s except for the occasional publication of pamphlets. Most provinces followed soon after; only Ontario kept up much of an effort.

The federal government once more became extensively involved during the Second World War, then largely withdrew, preferring to make financial contributions to provincial programs and organizations such as the Canadian Public Health Association or the Health League of Canada. Provincial governments in turn collaborated with community groups and public-health organizations. Whenever organizers turned their attention to schools, still other groups and institutions became involved, including school boards, teaching associations, and churches, most notably the Roman Catholic Church because of the separate Catholic school system. These bodies were reticent about sex education, as will be seen in section 6.3. As a result STD education from the 1920s through the 1960s was often unco-ordinated, sporadic, and underfunded.

Between 1968 and 1970 there was a general reorganization of the federal department, now called National Health and Welfare. It reflected the restructuring of health care that occurred with the introduction of a national health-insurance system.[25] Attention at the federal level shifted from active intervention to overall surveillance. Under the very general terms of the new plan the federal role included regulating the introduction of new drugs and the sale of all remedies; epidemiological analysis; other measures to protect the health of Canadians; measures to promote or maintain people's health, with a particular focus on lifestyles; financial support of provincial programs; and long-range health planning. The VD Division was absorbed into the Bureau of Communicable Disease Epidemiology in the Laboratory Centre for Disease Control. Ottawa no longer paid special attention to STD, and the burden fell more directly on the provinces.

Government response to AIDS was slow and at first not very substantial, particularly at the federal level.[26] Initially Ottawa tried to cope with the new disease through the Laboratory Centre for

Disease Control. A National Advisory Committee on AIDS was created in 1983. In 1986 the task was transferred from LCDC to a special office that in 1987 became the Federal Centre for AIDS (FCA). Action was hampered at first by small budgets, limited personnel, and an apparent reticence among key figures in government. Efforts focused on monitoring the epidemiological picture, testing drugs, and devising guidelines for the diagnosis, handling, and treatment of patients. In 1986 a national AIDS program was announced, along with a larger budget, but the plan remained a sketch. Critics pointed out that Ottawa still provided feeble leadership and avoided many recommended actions. In 1989 the FCA produced a five-point program that was a slightly revised version of the 1986 plan, still couched in very general terms, and thereafter said little more about its strategy. Most provincial and municipal governments dealt with AIDS through established divisions in their departments of health, with or without advisory committees.[27]

AIDS prompted the formation of far more local and community-based organizations than had previous STD crises.[28] Distrusting public authorities who in the past had been antipathetic towards them, gays set up their own organizations in major cities of all ten provinces, beginning in Vancouver, Montreal, and Toronto at the end of 1982 and the beginning of 1983. The first Canadian AIDS conference was held in 1985 to bring these groups together, exchange ideas, and plan strategy. There the Canadian AIDS Society was established as a permanent co-ordinating body. Frustration at government inaction prompted the formation of explicitly political organizations of AIDS activists such as AIDS Action Now (1988), which lobbied politicians and organized other forms of political pressure for better treatment of people with AIDS.

The same pattern as appeared in STD education recurred with AIDS. Government inaction drove community groups to develop their own education programs, focused largely on the gay community. Efforts aimed at the general public picked up in 1986, when municipal and provincial governments began work. The federal government at first relied on the Canadian Public Health Association, only becoming directly involved in the fall of 1987. Despite talk of a national AIDS education program, none was developed.

This recurrent lack of direction was due in part to the reticence of certain governments but also to the fragmentation of responsibility for health education across diverse levels of government and throughout communities. New action usually began in cities, was then adopted by provincial governments and, after a few years, by the federal government. The political structures of the public-health system, then, have been a central part of the problem with STD in Canada, ensuring that measures were frequently implemented in an attenuated form.

3.2 Funding

The costs of STD control have been borne by all three levels of Canadian government. Levels of funding have been influenced by several factors, including the wealth of individual governments, the state of the economy, and the epidemiological picture. Expenditure has been highest during "crises" (identified by a surge in incidence), as in 1916–24 or 1938–48.[29] Sources of funding have followed the rhythm of the federal-provincial see-saw. For example, the federal grant was terminated in 1931 as part of the austerity program of the new Conservative government, but provincial and municipal expenditures continued. In 1937 the government of British Columbia launched an ambitious program inspired by Surgeon-General Thomas Parran's new VD campaign in the United States. Other provinces began to revitalize their programs. In 1938 a new federal grant was introduced, but it was restricted to the provision of free drugs and therefore much smaller than the original federal grant. Wartime problems eventually prompted the federal government to introduce a new conditional grant to support STD measures in 1943. Total expenditures across all levels of government rose steeply in the 1940s. Thereafter allocations were pared down, settling at much lower levels during the 1950s and early 1960s.

With the implementation of a national health-insurance system in 1968 there was in theory universal access to health care, and funds for treatment were to follow automatically under the terms of the provincial medicare plans. Overall expenditures grew with the increased incidence of sexually transmitted disease in the 1970s and 1980s, but special allocations for STD control virtually vanished into the general funding arrangements.[30] This left government much less attuned to STD work.

The nature and magnitude of government response was also affected by the diversity of opinion within communities and politicians' need to satisfy a large and heterogeneous constituency. These considerations are reflected in the funds allotted to particular projects. Medical measures consumed most of the public funds throughout the twentieth century: the figure seldom dropped below 85 per cent of total STD allocations by federal and provincial governments.[31] Much less was spent directly on education, still less on "social services" such as contact tracing, patient counselling, and ensuring compliance with treatment until cured. Funding for STD research was always low.

The rising prevalence of AIDS prompted the reappearance of special allocations to cope with an STD.[32] In 1983, one year after the first case of AIDS was diagnosed in Canada, the federal government put $1.5 million over several years into research – a tiny sum that was soon increased by small increments. In May 1986 Ottawa finally committed $39 million over five years. For the first time the federal government allocated more money to education than to medical measures – the effect of limitations in treatment. In June 1988 $129 million was pledged for AIDS work over the next five years, including $30 million to medical care, $48 million to education, and $35 million to research – by far the largest support for STD research in decades. The sum was later raised to $168 million, but it was months before any funds actually made their way to those active in AIDS work.

The contributions of other levels of government varied considerably.[33] For a long time most provinces and municipalities incorporated expenditures on AIDS work into their general health budgets. In the summer of 1987 Ontario made a special allocation of $12.5 million to cover the next two years. At the same time Quebec came up with $2 million. In most of Canada responsibility for health measures with regard to STD rested to an important extent on municipalities. The bulk of AIDS cases were concentrated in Vancouver, Toronto, and Montreal. Toronto and Vancouver eventually provided substantial sums for their departments of public health. Indeed, Toronto had one of the largest budgets for AIDS work at any level of government. In July 1987 city council voted to spend $11 million over two years. Montreal was not in a position to supply similar levels of support because the province maintained a close control over health care and would not allow the city's proposal to redistribute tax funds.

4 · MEDICAL CARE

Canadian STD programs have placed heavy emphasis on medical care. That being the case, it is necessary to look briefly at the arrangements for its provision.

4.1 Diagnosis

There are actually very few "tests" for sexually transmitted diseases.[34] In 1906 the Wassermann test was introduced, which detects the presence in the blood of the specific antibodies formed by the body to eliminate the spirochetes that cause syphilis. The test was complicated, expensive, and occasionally inaccurate, but with time new tests improved detection. None, however, resolved the problem of the considerable cost. In the 1980s confirmation of herpes genitalis was made possible by the introduction of an enzyme immuno-assay test that detects the herpes antigen. Antigen-detection techniques for chlamydia were introduced in the mid-1980s but remain problematic. Thus, for NSU, chlamydia, and gonorrhea, detection still rests primarily on signs and symptoms, and identification of the causative organism by microscopic examination or culture. In 1983, two years after AIDS was first noted, the human immunodeficiency virus (HIV) was identified. The following year the enzyme-linked immunosorbent assay (ELISA) test was developed. ELISA works by identifying the antibody for HIV. Again, results were not always good: not only were there occasional false-positive results, but "false-negative" readings also occurred because those infected with HIV did not immediately develop detectable antibodies for the virus. Other tests have since been developed, and these can be used to corroborate ELISA results.[35]

4.2 Treatment

The twentieth century has been an era of "miracles" in medical science. We are therefore unaccustomed to think of the limitations of our remedies, even though they were and remain significant. One particularly significant limitation is the absence of effective vaccines for any of the sexually transmitted diseases. This places even more emphasis on treatment, which has always had important shortcomings.

Of the major sexually transmitted diseases, syphilis was not effectively treated until 1910, when Paul Ehrlich introduced arsphenamine, trade name Salvarsan. In several shots it was able to bring about a rapid cure for many cases, where earlier remedies required months and years of treatment, with no guarantee of a cure. Discovery of the drug, a complex organic compound containing arsenic, marked the beginning of a new era. Researchers now set out to find elaborate synthetic compounds that would have a specific action on particular disease-causing organisms. Salvarsan, however, had serious side-effects in some patients, and so doses had to be reduced and treatment prolonged.[36]

Another problem with the new chemotherapy was the expense. Large amounts of time and resources were required to develop a drug. Synthesizing the compound required elaborate equipment. This led to increasing dependence on large pharmaceutical firms for drug supplies and further therapeutic innovations. Their prices, however, reflected not only expenses but also the desire for a good profit. Drug costs therefore became an important element in the economics of disease control.

In 1943, soon after its discovery, penicillin was found to work rapidly against syphilis. As the first antibiotic it heralded a new class of agents that were even more efficient than Salvarsan. Penicillin, in one form or another, remained the treatment of choice from the 1940s to the 1990s.[37]

The treatment of gonorrhea and NSU went through two major changes in quick succession.[38] From the middle of the nineteenth century until the end of the 1930s all that could be done was to apply simple local antiseptics, usually solutions of silver nitrate or potassium permanganate. Patients had to return for many "washes" or "irrigations" – hardly pleasant procedures, and not especially effective ones, either. In 1936 another product of the chemotherapeutic revolution appeared: sulphanilamide, and in its train the "sulpha drugs." At last it seemed that there was a rapid, decisive cure for gonorrhea. Unfortunately, these drugs were seriously toxic and could prompt severe reactions. Worse still, the bacteria adapted to them with alarming rapidity. By the early 1940s there were several strains of sulpha-resistant gonococci.

Penicillin appeared to transform conditions, but soon there were problems. In the mid-1950s physicians found that the gonococcus was developing resistance to their new drug; doses had to be increased, and cures were not as rapid. Several newer antibiotics were used, notably erythromycin, spectinomycin, and tetracycline. Then a very disturbing discovery was made: certain strains of gonococci produced an enzyme that broke down antibiotics. The first cases of penicillinase-producing gonococci were reported in Canada in 1976, and in the 1980s strains of the bacterium developed a resistance to tetracycline and spectinomycin. Again medical measures were proving less than decisively effective.[39]

Physicians also had difficulty treating cases of NSU, particularly those infections that were later found to be caused by chlamydia. Penicillin was ineffective, and it was only with the introduction of other antibiotics, particularly erythromycin, tetracycline, and doxycycline, that infections could really be cleared up.[40]

We are still without a cure for herpes or AIDS. Indeed, finding a drug that acts specifically against any virus has proved to be very difficult. The situation with AIDS is complicated by the fact that the human immunodeficiency virus mutates rapidly. None the less, several drugs appeared in the late 1970s and 1980s that could diminish the pain and severity of herpes outbreaks.[41] In 1986, five years after AIDS was recognized, one drug had been developed that slowed the progress of the disease: azidothymidine (AZT, trade name Retrovir). Drugs were also developed to retard the progress of organisms that take advantage of the debilitated immune system.[42]

4.3 Drug Supply

One problem for government-supported STD care was the provision of drugs. The cost of compounds, and continued reliance on private firms for both research and production, led to repeated difficulties. In the 1910s, for instance, when the system came into being, the principal drug used against syphilis was Salvarsan, which was carefully protected by patents. These patents were held by a German firm, but during the First World War Canadian firms were granted licences to market a similar preparation. The price of the drug, whether from the original firm or its Canadian successors, was very high. The government of Ontario therefore set out to produce the drug itself. In response the Canadian firms reduced prices by as much as half. Between 1917 and 1919 there was a long dispute over the patent rights of private drug companies. It ended when the commissioner of patents in Ottawa reluctantly decided, in view of the serious public-health problem, to grant a restricted licence to the province. By then several foreign firms were selling the drug in Canada and the price had dropped further. Ten years later governments relied entirely on these firms.[43]

Supply was the initial problem when penicillin was introduced. Many early tests of the drug were actually performed in Canada, and so it was quickly approved. But Canada lacked production facilities. Under the Food and Drug Act the federal government fixed standards of quality and potency and defined methods for testing production of all drugs.[44] Only one laboratory in Canada could produce penicillin in anywhere near commercial quantities in 1943. For nearly two years, therefore, penicillin was strictly rationed, with most committed to the military. Penicillin was not automatically used against syphilis and gonorrhea. It was expensive, and some physicians and officials considered Salvarsan or sulpha drugs to be sufficient for many cases. Some provinces, including Ontario, did not assist in providing penicillin for STD clinics until as late as 1950.[45]

The supply of drugs again caused controversy during the 1980s with the appearance of AIDS. Several drugs appeared to reduce or retard the devastation of AIDS and its associated diseases. The most promising of these was AZT, although it had serious side-effects, it was far from a cure, and it was very expensive. Initially, Burroughs-Wellcome, who held the patent for the drug, were willing to supply it free of charge for eighteen months to those in clinical trials. In an unusual move aimed at assisting research to meet the terms of the Food and Drug Act, Ottawa provided $1 million, and the Federal Centre for AIDS initiated the mechanism for the clinical trials. In April 1987 Burroughs-Wellcome withdrew its original offer to supply AZT free of charge. Unless the drug were approved for clinical use in Canada, the company would allow no new patients in the clinical trials that were under way and would charge those already involved $1,000 a month. At the end of May 1987 Ottawa gave in and issued a "limited notice of compliance" for the company, thereby making the drug generally available for use in AIDS patients, and the provinces agreed to pay Burroughs-Wellcome for the drug on behalf of the patients in whom the immune-system damage had reached a critical point.[46]

People with AIDS and activists criticized the federal government severely for being slow to clear drugs that might be of benefit. The British Columbia Civil Liberties Association introduced the concept of "catastrophic rights": individuals with a terminal illness should have the right to use any remedy that they believe might be of some benefit to them as long as access to such treatment does not harm others. The federal department of health was not moved. Meanwhile, people with AIDS resorted to obtaining drugs secretly inside and outside the country. In September 1988 the federal department approved more drug trials. But by this time the trials themselves attracted criticism from activists. As many as half the people involved in a trial might be placed on a placebo rather than on the research compound, effectively leaving them without any form of treatment, either approved or experimental, for a considerable period of time.[47] Finally, in February 1989 the department suddenly announced that under the long-standing Emergency Drug Release Program, drugs that had not yet received clearance in Canada could be released on a case-by-case basis provided there was a "medical emergency" and existing therapy was ineffective. The costs, however, would have to be borne by the patient. At the same time, measures were adjusted so as to speed the approval of AIDS drugs for clinical trials.[48]

4.4 Arrangements for the Armed Forces

Treatment arrangements for the armed forces reveal both technical problems and social influences. During the First World War Canadian medical officers had to deal with an alarming incidence of sexually transmitted infections.[49] The number of patients quickly overwhelmed facilities in England, so a special annex was opened beside the principal Canadian forces hospital. By the autumn of 1916 there were so many cases that the medical corps decided to establish special hospitals for them. Separate arrangements again were made in the Second World War, when treatment was provided through both unit medical officers and hospitals. This was the result partly of a medical crisis and partly of a decision to make what seemed to be the best use of equipment and specialists. In 1943, however, "segregation" was abandoned in recognition of the fact that it stigmatized STD patients and, if anything, was a less efficient use of resources.[50]

During the Second World War a significant number of women were enlisted. STD measures for them reflected social influences more than biological differences.[51] Initially, female personnel with VD were discharged instead of being treated as men were. This reflected the lower value placed on womanpower and the perceived shortage of men for combat. Some officers also argued that discharging women would be less stigmatizing, given the potential for scandals inside the ranks; others argued the reverse. Medical officers resorted to transferring women under treatment to avoid problems. When the Canadian Women's Army Corps became an integral part of the army in March 1942, officials grudgingly recognized the servicewoman's equal right to treatment. One exception arose when penicillin first came into use. Despite the tenacity of gonorrhea in women, the drug was reserved for male personnel until June 1944.

4.5 Arrangements for the General Public

From 1919 onward, treatment provisions for the general public remained much the same across the country. The provincial venereal-disease acts specified the diseases involved, who could treat them, and what they could use. The legislation also gave "regular" practitioners a monopoly of health care in this area because it forbade others from treating STD or advertising and selling remedies, and backed the prohibition by stiff penalties.[52]

A central feature of Canadian programs has always been the local clinic where diagnosis and treatment would be provided free of charge to anyone who came in. Its location was relatively easy to find – for example, through discreet listings in telephone directories. These clinics were expected to transform conditions, but they met with limited success. Numerous studies revealed several reasons. Physical facilities were often rather unpleasant. Many clinics were

underfunded, understaffed, and overcrowded, while others, especially in periods of low incidence, were almost empty. Medical staff
were hard to attract, and most worked in clinics on a sessional or
part-time basis only. At the same time, many patients disliked the
idea of going somewhere special for STD problems. They were anxious about privacy and the confidentiality of records. The persistently negative view of STD in the community encouraged many to
seek the most discreet treatment, and that was in the office of a
physician in private practice.

In every decade the majority of patients preferred to go to a private
physician. Recognizing this, provinces assisted by providing drugs
at no charge to these patients. The introduction of public health
insurance made this route even easier, and in the 1970s and 1980s
three-quarters of all STD cases were treated privately.[53] The problem
was that many physicians screened, diagnosed, treated, reported,
and followed up STD inadequately. The connotations of STD meant
that some were reticent to suggest testing, especially to women, and
patients in turn were reluctant to be screened for STD. Instruction
on STD in medical schools was inadequate, and there was little opportunity to do specialist training in venereology in Canada.

The attitudes and actions of people with STD also affected the
results of measures aimed at reducing the prevalence of the diseases.
Many did not realize that they had an infection until the disease
had progressed for some time because there were no signs or they
did not recognize them. Some were slow to seek medical care even
once aware of their condition. They faced the stigma attached to the
infection, and many would have to contend with increasing social
divisions between age groups and between the dominant culture
and many subcultures. Physicians might be perceived to be aligned
with the moral establishment, and turning to them could mean critical judgments of lifestyle and attitudes. Not surprisingly, patient
compliance was difficult to ensure. Many people left before treatment was completed, usually when they were relieved of the symptoms. This was particularly serious in cases of tenacious infections
by drug-resistant organisms. Other patients were quickly re-
exposed.

Since 1919 provincial public-health laboratories have performed
tests free of charge on samples from anyone. Laboratories generally
operate near full capacity; resources have often been limited and
facilities strained, especially since the 1970s, with the rise in incidence of gonorrhea, chlamydia, and AIDS.

Health care for people with AIDS was affected by the level of
knowledge and attitudes of doctors, surgeons, nurses, and den-

tists.[54] The situation was not as serious in Canada as in the United States, where many refused to handle AIDS patients. Still, initial fear of contagion changed only gradually as it became apparent that standard precautions were sufficient. There were cases where AIDS patients were treated differently from others and care remained below what was accorded to others.

Those who became committed to AIDS work faced severe challenges. As the disease was new, there were inadequate numbers of doctors and nurses with special training. The biological complexity of the disease far exceeded that of any other STD, and the pace of therapeutic change was rapid. AIDS also led to repeated acute and severe illnesses, and was invariably fatal – two features that greatly increased the pressure on caregivers. Moreover, as a chronic illness with several debilitating manifestations, it required elements of primary and ambulatory care that were, and remain, underdeveloped. Then too, inadequate remuneration for the time and services required discouraged private practitioners from focusing on AIDS, and this increased the heavy load on hospitals and clinics.[55]

5. PUBLIC-HEALTH MEASURES

Over the century, Canadians have persevered with certain public-health measures and avoided others for as long as possible, regardless of the results produced by each. Experience revealed that the most effective were practical measures aimed at helping individuals to avoid infection, while regulations aimed at directing individual conduct could achieve only limited results. These lessons were learned slowly and often forgotten. People wanted to believe that certain measures would be effective and refused to accept those that appeared to undermine their own value-system. Social views could override medical considerations, and "effectiveness" was determined in part by the dictates of particular value-systems.

5.1 Regulating Conduct

The first attempts at regulating individual conduct were made by the armed forces. During the First World War soldiers who developed an infection had a portion of their pay deducted and were posted to unattractive duties or certain squads during the treatment period. These measures were stigmatizing and soon proved to be ineffectual. By 1918 they were generally abandoned. Yet when war broke out in 1939, the armed forces again tried stopping pay and assigning men to particular duties during treatment.[56] These measures were abandoned in 1942 because experience once more revealed that punishment inhibited treatment programs by discouraging men from coming forward and driving them to seek relief elsewhere. Experience in both wars thus underlined the fact that punitive measures were counter-productive.

A seemingly easy target were people who had sexual contact with members of the armed forces.[57] During the First World War, however, control of prostitution in Canada was generally much less vigorous than in American centres. In Britain the overwhelming number of infections prompted officers from the Canadian, Australian, and New Zealand expeditionary forces to press for tighter controls. The British were reluctant to take radical action. They remembered the nineteenth-century Contagious Diseases Acts, withdrawn after protests against the infringement of women's civil liberties.

There was no consistent assault on prostitution during the next war either. The most determined effort was made in Vancouver, where action began in 1937 as part of the revived vD campaign.[58] Military authorities considered Montreal and Quebec City the worst areas and deplored the lax attitudes of civilian authorities. But as one MP told the Commons in Ottawa, these conditions also arose because military personnel were concentrated in those cities before they proceeded to England and Europe. Eventually both Quebec and Montreal were prompted to close some of their brothels.[59] Still, surveys of sexual activity and levels of infection reveal that regulation failed to alter the conduct of either men or women significantly.

Regulating the conduct of civilians was far more controversial. Provincial legislation theoretically enabled authorities to compel a recalcitrant person to get treatment, but it was largely a dead letter. Provincial statutes also stipulated that anyone knowingly infecting another person was subject to fines or imprisonment, in line with the terms of the federal Criminal Code Amendment Act 1919. However, the law specified that individuals could not be convicted if they had "reasonable grounds" to believe they were not infected at the time the offence was alleged to have been committed, and no one could be convicted on the evidence of only one witness without corroboration. These qualifications made the section virtually unenforceable, and indeed no one was prosecuted under it for years. Finally, in 1985, it was struck from the books.[60]

5.2 Medical Examinations

During the First World War the military opted for routine examination of men – the famous "short-arm inspections" by medical officers. In Canada as in England routine inspection of prostitutes (the European strategy) would have raised a furor both over the invasion of individual rights and the facilitation of promiscuity. Inspection of men's penises apparently did not prompt such qualms. The same measures were adopted, though less rigorously, in the Second World War.[61]

The only measure that came close to regular inspection of civilians was the implementation of compulsory tests for syphilis at the time of marriage. British Columbia made this requirement in 1937, followed by the three prairie provinces in 1945 and 1946. The effect of this measure is uncertain, and all four provinces abandoned it between 1979 and 1988.[62]

Under the terms of the provincial VD or public-health acts, medical officers of health had the power to enter any building if they had reason to believe that someone there might be infected, and to compel those found to have VD to get treatment. Few MOHs were prepared to take such action, and there is little record of the use of this legislation in prosecutions against prostitutes.[63] Since the advent of the Charter of Rights in 1982, such invasive public-health measures would probably be struck down in any case.

5.3 Reporting and Contact Tracing

During the two world wars officers in Canada tried to trace contacts of infected individuals. They argued that since immunization was not possible, it was logical to go after sources of infection – a line of reasoning that influenced Canadian measures for decades. Contacts, however, were difficult to trace, due to limited information about partners and limited co-operation from civilian police. During the First World War officers learned that in Canada only one-third of the women involved were paid in any way for sex, and bona fide prostitutes accounted for only 10 per cent of all contacts. Medical officers concluded that it was better to target places where sexual contact took place. They pointed to bars, dance halls, hotels, and railway stations, but they glossed over one of the favourite pick-up places: public parks. In the Second World War the same measures produced much the same results. This time, however, it was discovered that fewer than 10 per cent of the women involved were paid for sex.[64]

Under the provincial VD acts, all cases of certain diseases were to be reported to the board or department of health.[65] This would provide epidemiological data that would enable officials to monitor disease patterns and plan accordingly. Records of tests almost always named the individual until the 1980s. This practice was defended on the grounds that it would ensure accuracy and facilitate tracking of those who did not co-operate with treatment regimens. A major reason, however, was that officials wanted to identity people who had contact with the individual and bring those with an infection to treatment. While such measures had been remarkably effective against diseases like diphteria and tuberculosis, the difficulties encountered by the military might have made people pause before applying them to STD. In practice, emphasis initially lay on treatment and education rather than "social work" and "police work." However, during and after the Second World War contact tracing became much more diligent and intrusive in certain provinces, notably Ontario and British Columbia, and this persisted into the 1950s. The shift may have been related to post-war prosperity – more resources were available for social work – greater confidence in treatment, and a more conservative outlook in society, which now favoured policing strategies. Limited results and a declining incidence of VD made contact tracing a target for budget-conscious governments in the later 1950s. The rise of STD in the 1960s prompted an expansion of tracing, and efforts persisted into the 1980s.

While in theory contact tracing should have been effective, in practice it was not: the number of cases brought to treatment was seldom substantial. Among the various reasons was the growing reliance on private practitioners, whose concern was the individual patient. Contact tracing was time-consuming and unremunerative, and threatened the principle of confidentiality. It could be perceived as punishment and discourage patients co-operation. Indeed, patients often were not forthcoming: some made false statements, and many were wary about discussing activities such as extramarital sex, prostitution, and homosexuality, which society had declared immoral or illegal. Casual contacts by definition did not include an exhange of identifying information. Some diseases had long latency periods with uncertain periods of infectivity. Finally, the whole operation was costly, time consuming, and fraught with the difficulties of co-ordinating many individuals and agencies.

Contact tracing was one of the most controversial measures adopted to control STD largely because of its direct relationship to the social ramifications of venereal infection. Critics maintained that aggressive contact tracing in a state-sponsored system discouraged those most in need of medical attention and might actually increase the risk of spreading infection. Contact tracing also infringed on civil liberties: it marked a significant invasion of privacy and a breach of confidential information about the health of a person. Government officials repeatedly offered assurances that medical records were confidential, but this principle was not always realized in practice. In 1980 the Krever Commission revealed that improper disclosure of medical information occurred with disconcerting frequency.[66] Although the Canadian Medical Association had come out in favour of non-nominal testing for STD in 1976,[67] government officials continued to reject proposals for anonymous testing.

AIDS was made reportable in most provinces in 1983. Some only required that persons with AIDS be reported, but during the decade an increasing number of provinces and territories required that anyone who was antibody positive but asymptomatic be reported as well. Mandatory testing was instituted for donations of blood, organs, and semen – instances in which other people were at immediate risk. Voluntary testing applied to the general public. Provisions varied among the provinces. Some provinces allowed the samples to be sent under a code or initials, but Manitoba, Saskatchewan, and Nova Scotia required the patient's name. Once a patient tested positive, all provinces initially wanted a report stipulating name, age, sex, and risk factors. Both physicians ordering the test and laboratories performing them were supposed to report positive results. Some provinces required physicians to see that infected people were counselled, partners were notified, and everyone who was infected received treatment.[68]

Almost at once, disputes arose over the arrangements for voluntary testing.[69] Critics stressed that extraordinary precautions were needed in view of the hostility among members of the general community towards homosexuals, IV drug users, and people with AIDS. Non-nominal testing was frequently urged by AIDS groups and eventually by the Canadian Medical Association, especially since the only real need for names was in a state-sponsored contact-tracing program. Advocates pointed to the United States, where the availability of anonymous tests in the late 1980s increased the number of people who determined their status. The assumption was that the great majority would take responsible measures if positive. Everyone recognized that there was a tension between protecting the individual and protecting the community. In the past, this tension had usually been resolved in favour of the community, using a rough utilitarian argument typical of public-health policy. The AIDS debate pitted those committed to the "right of privacy" against those who argued that people had a "right to know" if they had been exposed to a serious disease, and the fatal effects of AIDS meant that physicians and public-health officials had a "duty to warn." Moreover, without nominal reporting, some warned, there would be no way to monitor the few irresponsible individuals who knowingly put others at risk, cases of which had already made headlines in Canada.

The province of Quebec was the first to adopt anonymous testing, using special forms with code numbers. In other provinces some physicians simply refused to follow the regulations and did not report patients who tested positive. Others filed non-nominal reports with MOHs, and these officials acquiesced in the procedure. Most provincial governments were reluctant to provide anonymous testing: Ontario, British Columbia, and Alberta in particular were strongly committed to state-directed contact tracing. But in April 1990 Ontario finally agreed to a pilot study of anonymous testing.[70]

5.4 Preventive Measures

The army, faced with many cases of VD, was the first to look seriously at condoms as a preventive measure.[71] During the First World War a long debate dragged on among officers, members of the clergy, politicians, and some citizens. Opponents alleged that distributing condoms would appear to condone birth control and promiscuity. In the end the army decided not to issue condoms to the troops. By the Second World War the military was less willing to defer to public opinion. Studies had revealed the effectiveness of condoms; to reduce levels of infection, officers would have to make condoms available. At first condoms were rationed, but eventually they were simply given out free on demand. This was no small operation; as one MP told the House of Commons early in 1943, the government spent $165,000 on condoms for the armed forces at a time when the VD grant to the provinces, was all of $50,000.[72] As one report later noted, the vast number of condoms made it plain that promiscuity was "anything but exceptional."[73] However, female personnel did not receive condoms to put on their partners. The armed forces were still very much part of a society whose moral code placed greater reproach for promiscuity on women than on men.

Preventive measures among civilians were even more problematic. Condoms were not promoted until the 1970s (as shall be seen in section 6.2). Because of the severity of the problem and the limitations of available drugs, AIDS forced the issue to the fore. Condoms provided significant protection against transmission of HIV, but their association with contraception still made promotion of their use controversial. The Royal Society of Canada was asked by the federal Department of Health to advise on what measures ought to be taken against AIDS. The society's report, released in April 1988, recommended, among many things, that the preventive qualities of condoms be publicized and suggested distributing them free to prison inmates. Once again such proposals were criticized as facilitating precisely the kind of sexual activity that should be discouraged. The solicitor general rejected the proposals regarding inmates – "We don't permit ... homosexual activity in our prisons" – prompting some to wonder how much he knew about prison life.[74] No public action resulted, but several private groups began distributing condoms to people in high-risk groups. Finally, in September 1989 the government of Ontario took the unprecedented step of making condoms available in schools. As in other areas of public health, a crisis finally prompted a change in policy long rooted in moral considerations.

A less controversial preventive measure pioneered during the First World War was to make special provision for people to wash with a disinfectant soon after exposure. In 1916 the Canadian army began establishing places where men could go after having sex. These were known as "blue-light depots," in reference to the light burning outside as a discreet indication of their location and purpose. To allay criticism, they were officially referred to as "early-treatment centres," a name that suggested they were treating disease rather than preventing it. At the beginning of the Second World War these centres returned under a new euphemism, "early preventive treatment," this time equipped with a little green light outside the entrance. Such centres were not, however, set up for women. The effectiveness of washing remained uncertain. Moreover, as with the distribution of condoms, washing appeared to facilitate extramarital sex and promiscuity and was therefore bound to attract criticism from some. For these reasons the measure was never adopted outside military circles.[75]

Despite the possibility that STDs might be passed through donations of blood, semen, and organs, there was little screening before the 1980s. With the rise in fertility clinics, closer screening guidelines were adopted. Not long after AIDS was identified in 1981, it was found that people might be infected through transfusions of blood. In the spring of 1983 the United States Public Health Service and the Canadian Red Cross requested that high-risk groups not donate blood. With the development of the ELISA test in 1984 it was possible to screen all blood donations, but regular screening was not begun in Canada until November 1985. Similar procedures were adopted for semen and organs.[76]

The need to cope with the spread of AIDS among drug addicts prompted some to press for measures aimed at assuring that needles were "clean." In its special report the Royal Society of Canada proposed distributing sterile needles to addicts. This was condemned by some as equivalent to tolerating or even facilitating illegal drug use. Later in 1988 community groups and public-health officials in Toronto began programs encouraging drug users to sterilize needles. Despite prohibitions in the Criminal Code, some physicians in Montreal and Toronto began distributing needles to addicts, arguing that this was an essential public-health measure. Finally, after months of consideration and controversy, Vancouver, then Toronto and Montreal began needle programs in 1989.[77]

6. EDUCATION

The remarkable thing about STD is not how little it figured in public discourse during the twentieth century but how much. However, advice about what to do was shaped by moral code as well as medical fact. While educators set out to overcome some attitudes, they accepted certain assumptions about those who were infected, and this reinforced aspects of the social construction of STD. Moreover, the design of education programs was affected by concerns about offending the public. As a result, instead of reshaping public understanding, educators often sustained prevailing views on sexuality and STD.

6.1 The Military: Intense Efforts for a Captive Audience

The first efforts at government-sponsored sex education began during the First World War.[78] When Canada entered the war, no one had given VD education a thought, but the rapidly rising incidence of infection soon had officers scrambling to respond. Between 1915 and 1917 the Canadian Expeditionary Force evolved an increasingly elaborate program. Lectures, sometimes illustrated with slides, were the principal form of information, and were of two types. The first stressed hygiene and disease prevention. Men were given instruction on general hygiene first; then the discussion turned to keeping the penis clean, and thence to venereal disease. Soldiers were told that "every woman of easy virtue" was infected. "Abstinence" was the best way to avoid infection. Should men expose themselves, they must wash at once with the tubes of ointment given to them when they went on leave, and additional facilities were located in their medical officer's hut or at an early-treatment centre. The second type of lecture, introduced later, emphasized moral considerations. The speaker, invariably a medical officer, reminded the men that they were serving their country and VD undermined the war effort.

After briefly discussing the "sex instinct" and its purpose, he turned to "the responsibility of parenthood" and the importance of the family. "Chastity," he assured the troops, was possible for everyone; it was not unmanly, nor would it diminish a man's sexual powers. Promiscuity, however, could lead to infection, and with that he described the effects of venereal disease. Thereafter the men were treated to one type of lecture or the other according to what seemed to need emphasis – urging the men to be "continent" or telling the incontinent what to do.

During the Second World War the Canadian armed forces developed a program again relying on lectures and pamphlets.[79] The message was much the same as before, except that use of condoms was urged if the men were unable to abstain. They were ordered to report any infection but were assured that others would not know because records were strictly confidential.

Information for women was less explicit than for men and contained nothing on the use of condoms and disinfectant washes. Material stressed sexual abstinence and backed the message with the threat of serious social consequences for women who developed an infection. There was no emphasis on the confidentiality of records, and the general impression was created that any woman who developed an infection was bound to be perceived as "loose" and "unladylike." The army found it difficult to drop the lady/loose-woman dichotomy when dealing with female personnel because its program for men relied so heavily on it. Educational material for female personnel did not create a threatening male figure corresponding to the threatening female in literature for men, even though, with the rising incidence of vd, men could be seen as a threat to women both inside and outside the armed forces.

Case surveys revealed that military men picked women up because both freely wanted sex; "commercialized" sex with prostitutes was not common.[80] As officers saw it, this left them with the difficult task of making all "easy" women unattractive because they were potentially diseased. The problem with this approach was that it was so vague as to create negative stereotypes about a large part of the female population. A classic example was the pamphlet "Three Queens but I'll Pass," in which a series of cartoon figures depict gonorrhea and syphilis as women who can cause a man much harm. The same treatment reappeared in posters with captions like "He 'picked up' more than a girl."[81] This move to make women unattractive by associating them so closely with disease, besides being grotesque, was also a failure, since the positive appeals of sex and of women as persons was much stronger. After the war officials reported that "to attempt to reduce sexual promiscuity by the threat of venereal disease is certainly not getting at the root of the problem," and in any event "nothing we had to say influenced the sex habits of ... personnel very much."[82]

6.2 The General Public: Diffuse Efforts for a Large Audience

Education programs for the general public have been in existence since the First World War, but the results have been limited by wavering commitment, the methods employed, and the message presented.

"Campaigns." Efforts by governments and agencies were intense from about 1919 to 1924, and important ground-breaking work was done. Education programs across Canada declined markedly between 1925 and 1929, and remained limited during most of the 1930s. The field was largely left to the Canadian Social Hygiene Council, whose grants from governments actually rose until they were cut back in the early 1930s as part of the austerity measures brought on by the Depression. None the less, the cshc (later the Health League of Canada) was able to produce *Damaged Lives* in 1933–34, a feature-length film portraying the misadventures of a young man and the woman he went on to marry. The film was seen by hundreds of thousands in Canada and met with world-wide success.[83]

With the return of war, public-health officials recognized a need to intensify education programs. Yet little happened for three years. The Health League of Canada increased its work. British Columbia, the province most heavily committed to vd control at the time, strengthened its programs in 1940, and Quebec followed almost two years later. std education really revived when the federal government re-established its vd division in 1943. Between the end of 1943 and 1946 there was an unprecedented outpouring of material on sexually transmitted disease. Activity reached a peak in November and December 1944, when the government organized a "media blitz" involving newspapers, magazines, and radio. After the war the campaign lost momentum. The first indication came from the slump in articles appearing in papers and magazines during 1946. By 1949 it had fizzled out.[84]

During the 1950s and early 1960s astoundingly little was said or done by way of VD education in Canada.[85] There were extremely few articles on vd in newspapers, magazines, or even medical journals. The success of antibiotic therapy and declining rates of infection made it politically unnecessary and even controversial to have an information campaign. Paradoxically, medical capabilities made it easier to withhold knowledge.

In the 1960s Canadians discovered that drugs alone would not stop STD. The increasing incidence of infection prompted a more extensive approach to education on sex and STD, much as happened during the two world wars.[86] Education measures were intensified by the provinces and some community groups, as well as the Canadian Public Health Association in the later 1960s. From 1971 to 1973 there was an extensive education program in some provinces, notably Ontario. Once again, it ran for only a few years before losing momentum. There was another period of increased effort in 1977–78, especially in Ontario, Manitoba, and British Columbia. With the number of reported cases rising to very high levels by the early 1980s, yet another major effort was made, this time nation-wide, with the assistance of the federal government. This was overtaken by an even greater public-health problem – AIDS.

Because there was no vaccine, no cure for the disease, and no way to render patients non-infectious, the only means available to limit the spread of AIDS were preventive measures, notably avoiding certain practices and using appropriate mechanical barriers. These then had to be promoted by public education. However, an extensive education campaign was only slowly mounted, the effect of divided direction, initial uncertainty about the magnitude of the problem, limited knowledge about the disease in the early days, and negative attitudes towards gays. The federal and provincial governments did little from 1982 to 1986. The most innovative and constructive work in education was undertaken by community groups, which were active from 1983 onward. Several municipalities, notably Toronto and Vancouver, went ahead without waiting for the provincial and federal governments. Certain provinces, most notably Ontario, organized major campaigns, beginning in 1986, but efforts only became intense in the summer of 1987. The federal government finally became directly involved in the fall of 1987, but a national education plan to deal with AIDS was not developed.[87]

Methods. From 1919 to the present Canadians have employed the same basic educational devices and methods.[88] Pamphlets, the most common element, were produced by the federal government and some provinces as well as private organizations such as the CSHC/Health League of Canada and the Canadian Public Health Association. Articles and notices were run in newspapers and magazines, and more specialized pieces appeared in medical journals. Displays, some open, others enclosed, were set up at annual fairs in towns and cities, including the Canadian National Exhibition in Toronto and the Pacific National Exhibition in Vancouver. Posters were produced, as well as notices for public lavatories, bars, and similar places. Billboards were sometimes used, notably during the Second World War and in the AIDS campaigns of the later 1980s. Organizers also relied quite heavily on public lectures, frequently illustrated with slides and motion pictures. As early as the 1920s educators had experimented with feature-length films and shorter documentaries in both standard and animated forms. In the 1980s material also appeared in video form. By contrast, radio was used sparingly in every decade. Its strength was also its drawback: radio broadcasts could be picked up by anyone of either sex and any age, and so it was difficult to devise a program that would not offend someone. For the same reason, very little use was made of television. Broadcast information only increased in the 1980s. More discreet methods that responded to the particular needs of individuals were devised however. In 1971 the Ontario Department of Health began the first telephone hotline for STD information.[89] Such lines went into operation in many places, coming into prominence during the AIDS crisis.

The same problems kept recurring.[90] Material often received only limited distribution. Articles and notices in newspapers and magazines tended to be vague. Access to public displays was sometimes restricted and in any event limited to those who attended the fairs and were motivated to look at them. Posters presented only very general messages. Fitful use was made of other public notices. Audiences at lectures and film showings were usually segregated by sex from the 1920s through the 1940s, and the content for each was slightly different. Since anyone could receive radio and television broadcasts, discussion of STD remained very general, and even then networks might censor or reject material.[91]

A general problem with STD education was reaching the right people with the right information. Whereas the advertising industry had learned how to target sectors of the public, STD education rarely adopted its methods. Until the 1970s there were few attempts to focus on those groups most at risk of getting an infection. A series of bland or incomplete messages, confounded with moral postures, reached a limited and unselected part of the population with limited and carefully selected facts.

STD programs relied to a large extent on the voluntary efforts of people to inform themselves. The public had to choose to learn about the diseases, but getting the public to pay attention and take in the information was in itself a major challenge. The repugnant features of STD and the fear their existence generated often blocked communication. Media coverage, with its spectacular stories of "victims," heightened alarm without providing adequate information about the diseases and how to cope. Furthermore, like other segments of society, the media were influenced by moral considerations, the more so, in some ways, for being always in view.

The shortcomings of STD education were underlined by the AIDS crisis. There was not much candour until 1988. Posters and other government announcements told the public to inform themselves and indicated where they might find information, but provided few facts on the spot. In 1987 government radio notices told Canadians that AIDS was spread by "the exchange of body fluids" – a euphemism worthy of the Victorians. At the same time, huge posters showed pictures of (straight) couples or three men and a woman, simply to call attention to telephone hotlines. At the end of 1989 the Ontario government belatedly brought out posters with more direct messages, such as "You're sleeping with every partner your partner ever had. Cut the risk of AIDS; use a latex condom."[92]

Part of the problem was the persistent reticence of Canadians in general to accept candid discussions of sex and sexually transmitted disease. In 1987 the government-owned Canadian Broadcasting Corporation refused to broadcast notices on its television stations urging the use of condoms. Private companies, through the Canadian Association of Broadcasters, at first rejected AIDS announcements and then, in an elaborate public-relations manoeuvre, turned around and criticized government for not putting up money to pay broadcasters for air time. Most stations were not prepared to run AIDS notices as a public service. Canada had in effect censorship of vital public-health information by both a public corporation (the CBC) and private companies.[93]

Ultimately, more direct measures were attempted. In March 1988 the Ontario Department of Health sent every household in the province a pamphlet called *AIDS: Let's Talk.*[94] Translations were made into all the languages of the major minorities. But this was a one-time measure, and as before with STD, the coverage soon subsided.

Limited resources led people involved in education to focus on those most affected by the new disease – homosexual men. Much of the attention came from special organizations that worked largely outside traditional information networks. The most notable efforts, predictably, arose from the gay community itself. Protective measures were frankly discussed and ingenious means devised to make them more attractive. For example, the AIDS Committee of Toronto produced a frankly erotic poster with a photograph of two nearly naked men about to remove each other's underwear. Around the picture ran the caption "Take it off ... put it on," and beside the words was the image of a condom. This was followed at the end of 1988 and the beginning of 1989 by other posters and convenient pocket-sized pamphlets with attention-grabbing pictures and explicit texts. [95]

Content. The message of the educational programs was filtered through a moral screen; social considerations doubled with medical concerns to determine content. Material from the 1920s to the 1950s had certain basic features. [96] Pamphlets, lectures, and films provided discreet information about the diseases and went on to tell people that treatment was widely available free of charge. Information was sketchy and illustrations rare, although some lectures attempted to shock men by providing photographic illustrations of the lesions and other manifestations of the diseases. The old concept of pure and impure women persisted, and with it the assumption that women had a greater need for modesty and a greater potential for shame. [97] From the 1920s to the early 1960s it was common to have different pamphlets for men and women. Those for men were generally more explicit on both anatomy and the diseases.

When it came to the issue of safeguarding themselves, people were generally given one piece of advice: abstinence was the best way to avoid infection. Occasionally men might be warned against prostitutes or multiple sexual partners, especially those who were easily persuaded to have sex. Sexual activity with numerous partners did in fact increase the chances of becoming infected and then spreading the disease. To discuss this made sense, but the response of educators was to insist that people not have sex except with a spouse after marriage. That this was of limited use could have been predicted from the experience of the armed forces during both wars. In civilian circles, however, moral expectations were more intense. It took a long time before those involved in STD control – and the community as a whole – would realize that it was necessary to provide people with information that would help them live their chosen lives in a safer manner.

Modifications in content took place haltingly from the mid-1960s onward. Changes in behaviour and differences in expression of sexuality became so obvious that educators had to respond. Pamphlets from governments and private organizations became more explicit and were illustrated. Advice on how to prevent infection, however, was still limited and still emphasized avoidance of dangerous activities. Discussion of condoms appeared only in the later 1970s. Homosexuality was seldom mentioned until the 1980s except in material produced for the gay community.[98]

AIDS eventually toppled the delicate balancing act that educators were still performing. Candid information was presented in the gay community from 1983 onward. Sexual freedom had been one of the key features of gay liberation. Now it became vitally important to recognize that there was an associated risk. Given the sexual candour favoured in gay culture, information could be presented clearly, in a gay-positive light and in the language of the subculture – all features that improved communication. By contrast, patterns evident in the first sixty years of STD education for the general public repeated themselves during the 1980s. In *AIDS: Let's Talk* the first words of advice were the same as those the soldiers heard in the First World War: "Abstain from sex." But just as in 1916, educators realized that this would not suffice, and in carefully guarded tones they went on to explain other ways to reduce the risks of infection.

Results reflected deficiencies. Public awareness of AIDS was high; public knowledge remained low. Surveys in the later 1980s found that more than half of the population held erroneous beliefs about how contagious AIDS was, who might be infected, and how they might contract it. The change in conduct that AIDS education sought to produce was not much in evidence in the general community. Research revealed that few heterosexuals knew or followed safer-sex guidelines. Many Canadians, especially the young, continued to avoid using condoms. By contrast, gay men became among the best informed about the disease, and sexual practices changed markedly.[99]

6.3 Schools: Reticence before a Young Audience

A considerable improvement in knowledge about sex and sexually transmitted disease could have been developed through schools, where almost all individuals now learned a large part of the basic information they had about the world around them. But Canadians found it very difficult to accept that as soon as young people have the ability to be sexual, they should gain access to knowledge about sex. By rationing information, adults tried to retain a high level of control over the thoughts and conduct of the young. During the early years of the VD campaign, 1917 to 1925, some organizers wanted to extend their efforts to schools, but they faced strong opposition. Throughout the interwar years there was very little sex education in schools. Canadians considered sex to be a separate matter best entrusted to parents in the privacy of their homes. Educators then turned their efforts to the parents, who were often found to be ill-informed, in the hope that they would adequately instruct their children. This did not work, and those most likely to get infected, the sexually active young, remained poorly informed. [100]

In 1942 VD lectures were introduced in British Columbia schools, some accompanied by films. These were done by Health Department officials. Classes were segregated by sex, and instruction was limited to those sixteen and older. No other province followed this lead, though Ontario experimented with slightly expanded instruction. [101]

Introduction of sex education at the secondary-school level began in the later 1960s, notably in Ontario, Quebec, British Columbia, and Alberta. The programs were controversial and therefore limited in scope. [102] Many parents were wary: the information that might be imparted was considered by some to be potentially damaging to the moral order. Conservatives wanted to restore "traditional values" and stress "family life." For many the solution to the STD problem remained the same simple formula that had pervaded education since the 1920s: reduce promiscuity. During the 1970s and 1980s classes were often voluntary, the information inadequate. Very little was said about STD, and preventive techniques in particular were not discussed. A major stumbling block, as organizers across the country repeatedly discovered, was that the teachers themselves were not well-informed, and some were overtly uncomfortable about leading such classes. However, visiting specialists were seldom welcomed. In the 1980s ignorance about STD was still high among canadian youth, and education about sex and STD in schools remained deficient.

During 1987 AIDS became a topic of instruction in public schools in most parts of Canada. None the less, private schools, and Catholic school boards as a whole, hesitated to implement an AIDS program. Despite strong public support for such education, bitter disputes developed over what would be said to the students. In Ontario, for example, several courses outlines stressed abstinence as the best way to avoid AIDS and offered little other advice about how to prevent infection. Instead of responding to teenagers' feelings and preparing them for the real world, such programs endeavoured to extend the period of life without sex. Even where there was a co-operative atmosphere, organizers had to begin by teaching the teachers, among whom the level of knowledge about AIDS was low. As with the general public, awareness of AIDS among school children was high while knowledge remained low. [103]

CONCLUSION

During the twentieth century there has been a constant expectation that medical science would find ways to eliminate the diseases that threaten us and our ways of life. For decades Canadians have imagined that decisive treatments leading to rapid cures are possible, and with them problems such as STD should be resolved. Not surprisingly, government efforts to cope with sexually transmitted disease have concentrated heavily on medical measures. The dream of rapid, effective treatment for STD is revealing. Medical treatment would eliminate a host of biomedical, environmental, and social problems: the solution would be brief and decisive.

The failure to overcome the problem of STD despite medical measures stems from problems mentioned at the outset of this essay. The biological and medical challenges remain substantial, while the larger public-health program ultimately aimed at achieving not only medical but also social objectives. The goal may have been to make Canada safe for sex, but in most people's minds it was not to be just any kind of sex.

Government STD programs were often subject to constraints on financial, material, and human resources. While competing priorities accounted in part for these shortfalls, it is also evident that general attitudes about STD influenced the willingness of governments to commit resources to particular kinds of work. The effectiveness of STD measures was further diminished by the sheer administrative problems of co-ordinating any program involving many people over a large area. Other limitations grew out of the Canadian federal system, which made it necessary to mobilize political will at several different levels and contend with power struggles among jurisdictions.

Above all, Canadian organizers repeatedly failed to deal effectively with the social dimension of sexually transmitted diseases. Health education was hedged round with prohibitions on "sensitive" topics, so that for most of the century there was not much information about sexual needs and STD. This response, and the resulting restrictions on what information could be presented, played into the prevailing moral tenor of each decade, and led to misdirected promotion of abstinence as the key preventive measure.

In future STD programs must adjust to both biological and social factors. Medical capabilities will likely remain imperfect, and attitudinal changes occur through a slow process of dialogue between individuals and groups in a community. The most effective way to deal with STD is to adopt measures that are aimed directly at elimination of disease and are sensitive to human realities. This means frank acknowledgment of sexual diversity, epidemiologically based information, candid communication and education, and adequate medical facilities geared to the people involved.

NOTES

Abbreviations

CDWR: *Canada Diseases Weekly Report*
   CFP: *Canadian Family Physician*
   CGA: Canadian Gay Archives
   CJPH: *Canadian Journal of Public Health*
CMAJ: *Canadian Medical Association Journal*
     CN: *Canadian Nurse*
    GM: *Globe and Mail*, Toronto
   NAC: National Archives of Canada, Ottawa
     TS: *Toronto Star*
     PR: *La Presse*, Montréal
   UMC: *Union Médicale du Canada*

Research for this essay was undertaken during a post-doctoral fellowship at York University supported by the Social Sciences and Humanities Research Council. I also benefited from my position as archivist of the AIDS Committee of Toronto. I am grateful for helpful discussions with Dr Bruce Casselman, Ms Niki Cunningham, Mr Rob Elliott, Professor Susan Houston, Mr Ed Jackson, Dr Doug MacFadden, Dr David Naylor, Professor John O'Neill, Dr Samuel Solomon, and for assistance from Barbara Wilson at the NAC.

1 J. Cassel, *The Secret Plague: Venereal Disease in Canada, 1838–1939* (Toronto: University of Toronto Press 1987), chaps. 5 and 7.
2 J.E. Campbell, "Venereal Diseases," *CJPH* 17 (1926): 106–13; T. Parran, *Shadow on the Land* (New York 1937); J. Cleugh, *Secret Enemy: The Story of a Disease* (New York and London: Thames and Hudson 1954); T. Rosebury, *Microbes and Morals: The Strange Story of Venereal Disease* (New York: Viking 1971); S. Buckley and J.P. Dickin McGinnis, "Venereal Disease and Public Health Reform in Canada," *Canadian Historical Review* 63 (1982): 337–54.
3 E. Fee and D.M. Fox, eds., *AIDS: The Burdens of History* (Berkeley and Los Angeles: University of California Press 1988); D. Crimp, ed., *AIDS: Cultural Analysis, Cultural Activism* (Cambridge, Mass, and London: MIT Press 1988); S. Sontag, *AIDS and Its Metaphors* (New York:

Farrar, Strauss and Giroux 1988); R. Goldstein, "Bishop Berkeley's Virus: The Two Cultures of AIDS," *Village Voice,* 14 Mar. 1989, 49–51.

4 A.M. Brandt, *No Magic Bullet: A Social History of Venereal Disease Contol in the United States since 1880* (New York and Oxford: Oxford University Press 1985), 5, 6.

5 *Merck Manual,* 15th ed. (Rahway, NJ: Merck, Sharp and Dohme 1987); K.K. Holmes et al., *Sexually Transmitted Diseases* (New York, San Francisco, Toronto McGraw-Hill 1984); Institute of Medicine, *Mobilizing against AIDS,* 3rd ed. of *Confronting AIDS* (Cambridge and London: Harvard University Press 1989).

6 This section on attitudes to STD is generally based on Brandt, *No Magic Bullet;* Cassel, *Secret Plague;* D. Crimp, ed., *AIDS: Cultural Analysis, Cultural Activism;* Fee and Fox, eds., *The Burdens of History;* R.R. Pierson, "The Double Bind of the Double Standard: VD Control and the CWAC in World War II," *CHR* 62 (1981): 31–58; Sontag, *Illness as Metaphor* and *AIDS and Its Metaphors;* M. Rodway and M. Wright, *Decade of the Plague: The Sociopsychological Ramifications of Sexually Transmitted Diseases* (New York and London: Harrington Park Press 1988); J. Callwood, *Jim: A Life with AIDS* (Toronto: Lester & Orpen Dennys 1988); D. Spurgeon, *Understanding AIDS, A Canadian Strategy* (Toronto: Key Porter 1988); D. Helwig, "AIDS Tales: When Knowledge Is Scant or Conflicting, Folklore Takes Over," *CMAJ* 140 (1989): 1084–5.

  Canadian attitudes about STD are revealed, from certain perspectives, in the correspondence, lecture notes, pamphlets, and newspaper articles preserved in NAC, RG 29, boxes 207–10, 212–21, 493–7, 1234–6; MG 28 I 332: VD files, and CGA, Records of the AIDS Committee of Toronto. There are numerous articles in *CPF, CJPH, CMAJ, CN, UMC.*

7 Sontag, *Illness as Metaphor* and *AIDS and Its Metaphors;* Crimp ed., *AIDS Cultural Analysis, Cultural Activism;* Fee and Fox, *The Burdens of History;* J.W. Ross, "Ethics and the Language of AIDS," in C. Pierce et al., *AIDS Ethics and Public Policy* (Belmont: Wadsworth 1988).

8 On the history of sexuality, see J. Weeks, *Sex, Politics and Society: The Regulation of Sexuality since 1800,* 2nd ed. (London and New York: Longman 1990), and *Sexuality and Its Discontents* (London, Boston, and Henley: Routledge and Kegan Paul 1985); J. D'Emilio and E.B. Freedman, *Intimate Matters: A History of Sexuality in America* (New York: Harper and Row 1988); J. Costello, *Virtue under Fire: How World War II Changed Our Social and Sexual Attitudes* (Boston and Toronto: Little, Brown 1985); Cassel, *Secret Plague;* E.S. Herold, *Sexual Behaviour of Canadian Young People* (Toronto: Fitzhenry and Whiteside 1984).

9 J.W. Tice, A.H. Sellers, and R.M. Anderson, "Sources and Modes of Venereal Disease Infection in the Royal Canadian Air Force," *CMAJ* 51

(1944): 397–403; Tice, Sellers, Anderson, and W. Nichols, "Some Observations on Venereal Disease Control in the RCAF," *CJPH* 37 (1946): 43–56.

10 See essays by Ross and Kopelman in Pierce and Van de Veer, *AIDS Ethics and Public Policy*; also Brandt, *No Magic Bullet*; Cassel, *The Secret Plague*.

11 G. Kinsman, *The Regulation of Desire: Sexuality in Canada* (Montreal and New York: Black Rose Books 1987); E. Jackson and S. Persky, eds., *Flaunting It! A Decade of Gay Journalism from The Body Politic* (Toronto: Pink Triangle Press 1982); Weeks, *Sex Politics and Society*; Costello, *Virtue under Fire*, chap. 7; Gigeroff, *Sexual Deviations in the Criminal Law: Homosexual, Exhibitionistic and Pedophilic Offences in Canada* (1968); Anonymous, "Living with Homosexuality," *CMAJ* 86 (1962): 875–8; editorial and letter, *CMAJ* 87 (1962): 883–4, 517; R. Rancourt, "Homosexuality among Women," *CN* 63 (1967): 42–4; M. Brennan, "The Patient with Homosexual Problems," *CFP* 18 (1972): 58–61; D. Cappon, "The Homosexual Hoax: This Aberration Is Not A Right," *TS*, 10 Jan. 1973; C. Kuntz, "Homophobia: How Physicians Treat Homosexual Patients," *CFP* 28 (1982): 530–3; J.H. Gold, "Homosexuality: A Review," *CFP* 29 (1983): 521–4.

12 "Tough AIDS Activist Was Proud of His Battle to Regain Hospital Job," *TS*, 30 Dec. 1988; "Parents Fight AIDS Infected Teacher," *TS*, 11 Oct. 1987; Goodman, "The Trials of Eric Smith," *New Maritimes* (Sept/Oct 1988): 15–18; Canadian Human Rights Commission, *Policy on AIDS* (May 1988).

13 Cassel, *Secret Plague*, 17–21.

14 Ibid., 123.

15 Ibid., 201–5.

16 W.R. Feasby, ed., *Official History of the Canadian Medical Services, 1939–1945* (Ottawa: Queen's Printer 1953) 2:444–7, Tables 27–9. "The Venereal Disease Problem in the Canadian Army," NAC RG 24, file 60–4–19 (19), reel C 5048; "VD Control Epidemiology," RG 24, file 8994–3, reel C 5308; and "Statistics of VD," RG 24, box 12613, file 11HYG VD/8/2.

17 Health reports for Canada and the provinces; National Health and Welfare, *Venereal Diseases in Canada*, and *Sexually Transmitted Diseases in Canada, 1976*, app. E.

18 For example, NAC MG 28 I 53, reel C 9815, Dominion Council of Health Minutes, 48th meeting, Nov.–Dec. 1945.

19 See n 17.

20 For statistics and their interpretation, see annual Health Reports for Canada and the provinces; *VD in Canada*, later *STD in Canada*; periodic reports in *CDWR*; S.E. Acres and E.W.R. Best, "The Epidemiology of

Syphilis in Canada," *Modern Medicine in Canada* 19 (1964): 53–61; J.H. Smith, "New Problems with an Old Disease," *CN* 60 (1964): 1085–9; M. St Martin, "La syphilis, maladie d'hier et d'aujourd'hui," *UMC* 93 (1964): 1327–33; "Why the Increase in Venereal Disease?" *CN* 61 (1965): 520; J. Grandbois, "Syphilis: maladie d'actualité," *UMC* 95 (1966): 728–33; S.E. Acres and J.W. Davies, "Venereal Disease Problem in Canada," *CN* 67/7 (July 1971): 24–7; L.E. Roskovsky, "Reporting Incidence: A Legal Viewpoint," *CFP* 21 (1975): 91–5; F.R. Manuel, "Reporting Incidence: An Epidemiological Viewpoint," ibid., 99–103; A. Meltzer, "Sexually Transmitted Diseases," *CJPH* 70 (1979): 366–70; D. Lawee et al., "Herpes genitalis in Patients Attending a Clinic for Sexually Transmitted Diseases," *CFP* 29 (1983): 258–64; M. Steben and J. Yelle, "Sexually Transmitted Diseases and the Family Physician," *CFP* 29 (1983): 622–3; D. Delva, "Social Implications of Sexually Transmitted Diseases," *CFP* 29 (1983): 1933–6; A.G. Jessamine et al., "Epidemiology and Control of Sexually Transmitted Diseases," *CJPH* 74 (1983): 163–6; J.C. Hockin and A.G. Jessamine, "Trends in Ectopic Pregnancy in Canada," *CMAJ* 131 (1984): 737–40; "Trends in Rates of Reported Gonococcal Infections in Canada, 1962–1983," *CMAJ* 132 (1985): 941–2; "Laboratory Reports of Herpesvirus Infections in Canada [1978–85], *CMAJ* 135 (1986): 1377–9; M. Todd et al., "Sexually Transmitted Diseases in Canada: An Overview," *CFP* 33 (1987): 1771–6; F.P. Scapatura, "Genital Herpes," *CFP* 33 (1987): 1835; "50% of Teen Prostitutes Carry a Sexually Transmitted Disease," *TS*, 5 Nov. 1987; "Chlamydia Now Communicable Disease," *GM*, 8 Nov. 1988.

21 B. Kanee and C.L. Hunt, "Homosexuality as a Source of Venereal Disease," *CMAJ* 65 (1951): 138–40; A.A. Larsen, "The Transmission of Venereal Disease through Homosexual Practices," *CMAJ* 80 (1959): 22–5; Toronto Department of Public Health, *Annual Statement* 1961, 55–6; Ontario, *Health Report* 1960, 32 and 1961, 32; C.C. Jackson, "The Venereal Esoteric," *CMAJ* 87 (1962), and "Anorectal Venereal Disease," *CFP* 15 (1969): 27–30; Grandbois, "Syphilis" (1966), 731–2; H.K. Kennedy, "The Control of Venereal Disease in British Columbia," *CJPH* 60 (1969); T.W. Austin, "Gonorrhea in Homosexual Men," *CMAJ* 119 (1978): 731–2; "Homosexual Men Prone to VD Survey Shows," *TS*, 3 Sept. 1981; S.J. Landis, "Sexually Transmitted Diseases among Homosexuals," *CMAJ* 130 (1984): 370–2, and J.C. Katz, letter, 131 (1984): 841; E. Domovitch, "A Comprehensive Approach to Male Homosexual Disorders," *CFP* 31 (1985): 1971–5; C.L. Soskolne et al., "Characteristics of a Male Homosexual/Bisexual Study Population in Toronto, Canada," *CJPH* 77 (1986): 12–16; B.C. Willoughby, "Health Concerns for Male Homosexual Patients," *CFP* 34 (1988): 1765–9. There was no discussion of lesbians and STD.

22 *Canada Diseases Weekly Report* 14/28, 16 July 1988; 15/10, 11 Mar 1989; 15/52, 30 Dec 1989; 16/9, 3 Mar 1990. Several cases have been retrospectively diagnosed for the period 1979–81.

23 Cassel, *Secret Plague*, 168–70, 199; Canada, Commons, *Debates* 1943, 344, 3176–9; 1944, 608–9, 3025–8, 3031–2; Canada, *Health Report* 1943–44, 60–1; D.H. Williams, "Canada's National Health and Venereal Disease Control," *CJPH* 34 (1943): 262–6; "A National VD Control Conference," *CJPH* 34 (1943): 575–7; Dominion Council of Health Minutes, 44th meeting, 30–1 Mar. 1943, NAC reel C 9815; NAC RG 29, box 213, file 311–V3–12, and boxes 493–7 file 311–V3–29.

24 *Health Reports* of Canada and the provinces; VD files of the Health League of Canada in NAC MG 28 I 332. Cassel, *Secret Plague*, 170–2, 206–45.

25 National Health and Welfare, *Annual Reports*, 1968–1974; M. Lalonde, *A New Perspective on the Health of Canadians* (Ottawa: National Health and Welfare 1974); D.D. Gelman, R. Lachaine, and M.M. Law, "The Canadian Approach to Health Policies and Programs," *Preventive Medicine* 6 (1977): 265–75.

26 National/Federal Centre for AIDS, *Annual Reports*; "Ottawa Called Negligent for Inaction on AIDS," *TS*, 17 May 1988; "Ottawa's Delays Stall the Fight against AIDS," *TS*, 1 June 1988; "Ottawa 'Doing Nothing' about AIDS, Critics Say," *TS*, 16 Jan. 1989; "Ottawa Announces First AIDS Policy," *TS*, 13 Apr. 1989; "Canada's Fight against AIDS Failing Miserably," *TS*, 16 Apr. 1989; Canada, Health and Welfare, *AIDS in Canada: The Federal Government Responds* (1989), *A Policy Framework for the Federal AIDS Program* (1989), and *AIDS Community Action Program*; "Ottawa Mum on Strategy to Combat AIDS," GM 28 Nov. 1989.

27 "City Health Department Programs," National AIDS Conference, 17 May 1988; Ontario, Ministry of Health, *Working Conference on AIDS and HIV Infection, December 1–2 1988, Summary Report.*

28 CGA, ACT Records, and 91–111, files on organizations; Health and Welfare Canada, *A Guide for Voluntary Human Service Organizations* (May 1989); Canadian AIDS Society, organization listings; *AIDS Action News!* 1 (1988) onward; *Le Manifeste de Montréal* (June 1989).

29 Health reports, annual estimates, and public accounts of Canada and the provinces; Cassel, *Secret Plague*, 194–201, app. D, E; Dominion Council of Health Minutes, 1938, 1943–49, 1952–53, 1954–55, 1959–62, reels C 9815–7; NAC RG 29, boxes 361–371A, 1409, files on VD and National Health Grants.

30 Canada, Statutes, *Medical Care Act*, 15 Eliz. II Ch 64, 1966–67; *Health Resources Fund Act*, 15 Eliz. II Ch 42, 1966–67; *Federal-Provincial Fiscal Arrangements Act*, 15 Eliz. II Ch 89, 1966–67, replaced by 21 Eliz. II Ch 8, 1972, replaced by *Established Programs Financing Act*, 25–6 Eliz. II

Ch 10, 1977. All replaced by *Canada Health Act,* 32–3 Eliz. ii Ch 6, 1984. Some details are in grants files in NAC RG 29, Acc 81–2/087 and VD; Acc 85–86/235.

31 In addition to n 29, see A.R. Ronald et al, "Research on Sexually Transmitted Diseases in Canada," *CJPH* 74 (1983): 173–5.

32 M.A. Wainberg and S.E. Read, "Public Funding for AIDS Research in Canada and the USA," *CMAJ* 134 (1984): 109–10; Federal Centre for AIDS, Annual Reports; Royal Society of Canada, *AIDS: A Perspective for Canadians* (Ottawa: RSC 1988): 26–8; "Cash Plea Ends AIDS Conference," *TS,* 19 May 1988; "Epp Pledges $129 Million in AIDS Fight," *GM,* 9 June 1988; "Beatty Vows Commitment to AIDS Fight," *TS,* 14 Apr. 1989.

33 "$12.5 Million to be Spent in AIDS Fight" and "Quebec Earmarks $2 million for AIDS," *TS,* 26 Aug. 1987; "Ontario Boosts Funding for AIDS," *TS,* 30 May 1989; "Toronto Okays $11 Million Plan," *TS,* 14 July 1987; "City Health Department Programs," National AIDS Conference, 17 May 1988.

34 Cassel, *Secret Plague,* 32–3; Holmes et al., *Sexually Transmitted Diseases,* chaps. 29–31; J.A. Geddes, "Interpreting Serological Tests for Syphilis," *CFP* 33 (1987): 1829–32; Canada, Department of Health and Welfare, *1989 Canadian Guidelines for the Diagnosis and Management of Sexually Transmitted Diseases.*

35 G.P. Wormser et al., eds., *AIDS and the Manifestations of HIV Infection* (Park Ridge, NJ: Noyes 1987), chap. 14; "The Significance and Accuracy of ELISA Tests," *CDWR* 13/1, 10 Jan. 1987; J.W. Frank et al., "A Critical Look at HIV-Antibody Tests," *CFP* 33 (1987): 2005–11.

36 Cassel, *Secret Plague,* chap. 3.

37 J.E. Moore, *Penicillin in Syphilis* (Springfield, Ill., and Toronto: C.C. Thomas and Ryerson 1946); Holmes et al., *Sexually Transmitted Diseases,* chaps. 29–31, 34–5; Health and Welfare Canada, *1988 Guidelines for the Treatment of Sexually Transmitted Diseases.*

38 Cassel, *Secret Plague,* chap. 3; T. Sollmann, *A Manual of Pharmacology,* 6th and 7th eds. (Philadelphia and London: W.B. Saunders, 1942, 1948); Holmes et al., *Sexually Transmitted Diseases,* chaps. 18–25; *1988 Guidelines for Treatment.*

39 E. Snell et al., "Susceptibility of N. gonorrhoeae to Antibiotics," *CMAJ* 89 (1963): 601–6; H. Dillenberg, "Problems in the Diagnosis, Treatment and Prevention of Gonorrhea," *CJPH* 55 (1964): 233–6; C.R. Amies, "Development of Resistence of Gonococci to Penicillin," *CMAJ* 96 (1967): 33–5; H.G. Robson and I.E. Salit, "Susceptibility of N. gonorrhoeae to Seven Antibiotics in Vitro," *CMAJ* 107 (1972): 959–62; J.R. Dillon et al., "Penicillinase-Producing N. gonorrhoeae in Canada," *CMAJ* 125 (1981): 851–5; "Tetracycline-Resistent N. gonorrhoeae (TRNG) – Ontario," *CDWR* 13/34, 29 Aug. 1987; "High Rates of Penicil-

linase-Producing N. gonorrhoeae Strains – Quebec," *CDWR* 14/49, 10 Dec. 1988; "Emergence of Spectinomycin-Resistent Strains of N. gonorrhoeae in Quebec," *CDWR* 15/19, 13 May 1989; "MDs Urged Not To Use Penicillin, Tetracycline to Treat Gonorrhea," *GM*, 4 May 1990.

40 Holmes et al., *Sexually Transmitted Diseases; 1988 Guidelines for Treatment*.

41 Holmes et al., *Sexually Transmitted Diseases*, chaps. 42–3; F.P. Scappatura, "Genital Herpes," *CFP* 33 (1987): 1835–9; *1988 Guidelines for Treatment*.

42 R. Yarchoan et al., "*AIDS* Therapies," *Scientific American* 259 (Oct. 1988): 110–19; *1988 Guidelines for Treatment*; Institute of Medicine, *Mobilizing against AIDS*; C. Farber, "Sins of Omission: The *AZT* Scandal," *Christopher Street* 12 (1989): 9–14.

43 Cassel, *Secret Plague*, 151–3, 164–7.

44 Health and Welfare Canada, *Food and Drug Regulations*, esp. sec. C.08; *Guidelines for Preparing and Filing New Drug Submissions*.

45 "Toronto Studies on Penicillin," *CMAJ* 49 (1943): 422–3; "The Supply of Penicillin," *CMAJ* 50 (1944): 457; "Penicillin for Civilian Use," *CMAJ* 51 (1944): 172; "The Manufacture of Penicillin," ibid., 467–8; "Penicillin and Venereal Diseases," *CMAJ* 52 (1945): 508; "Government Control of Penicillin Relaxed," ibid., 287; Dominion Council of Health Minutes, 1944–47, NAC reels C 9815–6; "Urges Province Provide Penicillin To Combat VD," *GM*, 13 June 1950.

46 "Approval of New Drug for AIDS Is Urged," *TS*, 14 Apr. 1987; "Accord Reached To Expand Use of Anti-AIDS Drug," *TS*, 23 May 1987; Cohen, "Federal Centre"; Health Protection Branch, Health and Welfare Canada, circular letters ("Issues") on AZT trials, 10 and 18 Aug. 1989.

47 AIDS Action Now, *Treatment AIDS!, AIDS Action News!* 1 (1988–present); "Advocacy Action on AIDS," *NOW* magazine, 28 Jan.–3 Feb 1988; "Unapproved AIDS Drugs Reported Used in Hospice," *TS*, 20 May 1988; "Inaccessible Drug Therapies Infuriate People with AIDS," *NOW*, 11–24 Aug. 1988; "AIDS Group Protests Placebo Tests," *TS*, 16 Sept. 1988; "Marchers Protest Lack of Drugs," *TS*, 23 Oct. 1988; Ontario, *Working Conference on AIDS, December 1988*, 16–24.

48 "Drugs for the Treatment of AIDS," circular letter from Health Protection Branch, Health and Welfare Canada, 8 Feb. 1989; "Victory for Life," *Xtra*, 10 Feb. 1989; "Canada Helping Its Critically Ill Obtain Any Drug, Even If It Is Unapproved," *New York Times*, 26 Feb. 1989.

49 The principal records for the military VD program in the First World War are NAC RG 9, ser. III B2, file 25–11–1 (1–12), and RG 24, file 60–4–19. See also Cassel, *Secret Plague*, chap. 6.

50 The principal records for programs in the Second World War are

NAC RG 24, boxes 6617–8, file HQ 8994–6; box 12612, file 11HYG
VD/7/3; boxes 15645–6 (war diary, DMS, CMHQ); file HQC 8328–614,
reel C 4986; file HQC 60–4–19, reels C 5048–9; Dominion Council of
Health Minutes 1939–46, reels C 9815–6. Ontario, Department of
Health, *Proceedings of the Venereal Disease Conference, October 10 1939*;
J.W. Tice et al., "Sources and Modes of Venereal Disease Infection in
the Royal Canadian Air Force," *CMAJ* 51 (1944): 397–403; Tice et al.,
"Some Observations on Venereal Disease Control in the RCAF," *CJPH*
37 (1946): 43–56. See also W.R. Feasby, ed., *Official History, 1939–1945*
2, chap. 7.

51 R.R. Pierson, "The Double Bind of the Double Standard: VD Control
and the CWAC in World War II," *CHR* 62 (1981): 31–58. In addition to
sources in n 50 see NAC RG 24, file HQC 8994–12, reel C 5318.

52 Cassel, *Secret Plague*, chap. 8 (for 1919–39); NAC RG 29, box 213,
file 311–V3–12, voxes 493–7, file 311–V3–29, boxes 497–8, file 311–V3–
30; Dominion Council of Health Minutes; Health Reports of Canada
and the provinces; G. Bates, "The Venereal Disease Clinic," *CJPH* 19
(1928): 466–72; R.P. Vivian, "The Public Health Aspects of Venereal
Disease Control," *CJPH* 36 (1945): 53–7; A.F. Chaisson, "Experience of
the New Brunswick Department of Health in the Control and Treatment of Syphilis," *CJPH* 44 (1953): 90–4; A.F.W. Peart, "The Venereal
Disease Problem in Canada," ibid., 160–6; W.I. Bent, "Problems in
Venereal Disease Control as Seen by a Medical Officer of Health,"
CJPH 56 (1965): 137–9; W.G. Allanach," ... as Seen by a Private Practitioner," ibid., 140–1; E.A. Robertson, "... as seen by a Public Health
Nurse," ibid., 142–3; H.K. Kennedy, "The Control of Venereal Disease
in British Columbia," *CJPH* 60 (1969); S.E. Acres and J.W. Davies, "Ve-
nereal Disease Problem in Canada," *CN* 67 (1971): 24–7; "The Nurse
and Venereal Disease Control," ibid., 28–30; J.D. Wallace, "It's Bad
Medicine – Legally and Morally," *CMAJ* 109 (1973): 776; "Govt.,
Profession Urge MDs to Provide Better Care," *CN* 70, no. 4 (Apr. 1974):
15; R.W. Mitchell, "Patients' Compliance with Follow Up after Treat-
ment of Genococcal Urethritis," *CMAJ* 116 (1977): 48–50; A. Meltzer,
"Sexually Transmitted Diseases in Canada," *CJPH* 70 (1979): 366–70;
L.E. and F.A. Roskovsky, "Sexually Transmitted Diseases and the
Law," *CJPH* 74 (1983): 135–6; D. Delva, "Social Implications of Sexually Transmitted Diseases," *CFP* 29 (1983): 1933–6; B. Romanowski,
"Sexually Transmitted Diseases: A Time for Action," *CJPH* 74 (1983):
153–4; S.L. Sacks et al., "Education and Public Awareness of Sexually
Transmitted Diseases," ibid., 176–8; A.A. Adrien et J. Carsley, "Éléments d'un programme régional de contrôle et de prévention des MTS
dans la région de Montréal," *UMC* 115 (1986): 519–21; STD issue, *CFP*
33, no. 8 (Aug. 1987).

53 Meltzer, "STD in Canada," 367; M. Steben and J. Yelle, "Sexually

Transmitted Diseases and the Family Physician," *CFP* 29 (1983): 623.
54 Hospital staff and physicians: I. Mackie, "AIDS and Organized Medicine: Our Profession Has Failed To Lead," *CMAJ* 138 (1988): 560–1, and letters, ibid., 1083–4; RSC, *AIDS*; discussions at National AIDS Conference, May 1988; "Fear Leads to AIDS Patients' Isolation," *TS*, 27 Sept. 1987; "Hospitals Told To Tighten Protective AIDS Measures," *TS*, 21 June 1988; "AIDS and Nurses: A Knowledge Gap," *TS*, 17 Aug. 1988; "Nurses Confused by AIDS," *GM*, 29 Sept. 1988; "Precautions Can Handle AIDS Virus Risk," *GM*, 24 Sept. 1988; "Gay Patient Angered by AIDS Warning Card," *GM*, 22 Oct. 1988. Personal communications: participants in the Talking Sex Project, Toronto, 1988; Dr David Naylor, Toronto, Dec. 1988; Dr Doug MacFadden, Toronto, Apr. 1989; Dr Samuel Solomon, Montreal, 7 June 1989. Canada, Department of Health and Welfare, *Recommendations for Prevention of HIV Transmission in Health Care Settings*.

Dentists: G.R. Thordarson, "Moral and Ethical Issues Related to Infectious Diseases," *Canadian Dental Assn Jnl* 53 (1987): 677–8; J. Hardie, "Dentists' Attitudes towards AIDS," ibid., 823–5; T. Tremayne Lloyd, "Dentistry, the Law and AIDS," ibid., 54 (1988): 407–8; T.D. Daley, "AIDS Risk and Dental Personnel," ibid., 825–7; "Dentists' Fear of AIDS Called Needless," *TS*, 8 Dec. 1988.
55 National AIDS Conference, Toronto, 16–17 May 1988; Ontario Ministry of Health, *Working Conference on AIDS* (Dec. 1988).
56 See nn 49, 50.
57 G. Bates et al., "Social Aspects of the Venereal Disease Problem," *CJPH* 8 (1917): 287–91; Cassel, *Secret Plague*, 123–4, 126–7, 142.
58 D.H. Williams, "Commercialized Prostitution and Venereal Disease Control," *CJPH* 31 (1940): 461–72, and "The Facilitation Process and Venereal Disease Control," *CN* 40 (1944): 89–96; W. Mulligan, "Cooperation by the Police in Venereal Disease Control," NAC RG 29, vol. 1234, file 311–V2–3 (2).
59 Canada, Commons, *Debates*, 1944, 593–4, 963; "Hits VD Link with Montreal," *GM*, 12 Feb. 1944; "Quebec City Jails Prostitutes," *GM*, 12 Oct. 1944; "Montreal Record Disgrace – Houde," *TS*, 6 Feb. 1945; "Round-Up 200 in Vice Blitz at Montreal," *Toronto Telegraph*, 19 Feb. 1945; "Most Venereal Disease Acquired in Montreal," *Telegraph*, 25 Feb. 1945; "Women Jailed in VD Round-Up," *GM*, 7 Mar. 1945. Little was said in the French Canadian press.
60 Roskovsky, "STD and the Law."
61 See nn 49, 50.
62 H. Orr, "The Compulsory Premarital Serological Test in Alberta," *CJPH* 38 (1947): 232–5; NAC RG 39, boxes 500 and 1239, file 311–V3–32.
63 NAC RG 29, boxes 206–7, file 311–V3–2; Roskovsky, "STD and the Law".

64 See n 57, and Tice et al., "Source and Modes" and "Some Observations"; NAC RG 24, box 12611, 11 HYG VD/2/5; RG 29, box 206, file 311–V3–2.

65 The following discussion is based on NAC RG 29, box 206, file 311–V3–2, and boxes 499–500, file 311–V3–31; provincial Health Reports; Toronto Department of Public Health, *Annual Statements*, espec. 1955, pp 54, 56; "More Regard [for] Enforcement of Control Laws Asked," GM, 10 Dec. 1943; Williams, "Facilitation Process"; E. Lalande and J. Archambault, "Administration of a Provincial Venereal Disease Control Program," CJPH 35 (1944): 55–9; G. Choquette, "Quelques aspects du service médico-social à la division des maladies vénériennes," UMC 73 (1944): 1195–8; C.A. Bourdon, "Contribution du Service de Santé dans la lutte antivénérienne à Montréal," UMC 76 (1947): 470–5; W.G. Brown and W.B. Nichols, "Epidemiologic Procedures as a Case Finding Mechanism in Syphilis Control," CJPH 39 (1948): 123–30; Chief Constables' Association of Canada, *1948 Convention*, 55–6; W. Mulligan, "Cooperation by the Police in VD Control," NAC RG 29, box 209, file 311–V3–3 (6); B.D.B. Layton, "The Practising Physician and the Control of Syphilis," CMAJ 63 (1950): 436–40; E.W. Thomas, "Problems in the Future Control of Syphilis," CJPH 42 (1951): 451–4; Peart, "VD Problem in Canada"; D.O. Anderson and A.J. Nelson, "Observations on the Applied Epidemiology of Gonorrhea," CJPH 45 (1954): 381–91; A.A. Larsen and W.J. Cunningham, "Venereal Disease Facilitation in Vancouver," CJPH 51 (1960): 49–56; Wallace, "Bad Medicine"; "CMA Board Considers Legal Side of VD Control," CMAJ 112 (1975): 751–2; Meltzer, "STD in Canada," 368; Roskovsky, "STD and the Law"; D. Delva, "Social Implications of Sexually Transmitted Diseases," CFP 29 (1983): 1934; J.K. Andrus, "Partner Notification – Can It Control Epidemic Syphilis?" *Annals of Internal Medicine* 112 (1990): 539–43. See also Cassel, *Secret Plague*, 188–90.

66 Ontario, *Report of the Commission of Inquiry into the Confidentiality of Health Information* (1980).

67 J.S. Bennett, "Sexually Transmitted Disease," CMAJ 117 (1977): 209.

68 Ontario, *Working Conference on AIDS, December 1988*, 25–38; D.G. Casswell, "Disclosure by a Physician of AIDS Related Patient Information: An Ethical and Legal Dilemma," *Canadian Bar Review* 68 (1989): 225–58; W.F. Flanagan, "Equality Rights for People With AIDS: Mandatory Reporting of HIV Infection and Contact Tracing," *McGill Law Journal* 34 (1989): 530–602; J. Hamblin and M.A. Somerville, "Surveillance and Reporting of HIV Infection and AIDS in Canada: Ethics and Law," *University of Toronto Law Journal* 41 (1991): 224–46.

69 In addition to the above, see "Anonymity Urged for Those Found with Link to AIDS," TS, 24 Oct. 1985; "Only Anonymous AIDS Testing Will Work," TS, 4 Jan. 1989; "A CMA Position: AIDS," CMAJ 140

(1989): 64A; "HIV Antibody Testing in Canada, Recommendations of NACAIDS," *CDWR* 15/8. 25 Feb. 1989; "City Approves Anonymous AIDS Tests," *Xtra*, 12 May 1989; AAN, *Testing AIDS* (May 1989); "Shared Test Results Vex AIDS Doctors," *NOW* 7–13 Dec. 1989.

70 "Anonymous AIDS Tests Okayed," *TS*, 17 Apr. 1990.

71 Cassel, *Secret Plague*, chap. 6; Pierson, "Double Bind."

72 Canada, Commons, *Debates* 1943, 344.

73 Tice et al., "Some Observations," 53.

74 Royal Society of Canada, *AIDS: A perspective for Canadians* (Ottawa: RSC 1988); "Inmates Should Get Free Condom Supply AIDS Study Says," *TS*, 28 Apr. 1988.

75 See nn 49, 50.

76 "AIDS and the Use of Blood Components and Derivatives: The Canadian Perspective," *CMAJ* 131 (1984): 20–2; "Anti-HIV Screening in Canadian Blood Donors," *CMAJ* 135 (1986): 901; N.A. Buskard, "Infectious Complications of Blood Transfusion," *CFP* 33 (1987): 1223–7; "Blood Supplies More at Risk from AIDS Researchers Say," *TS*, 16 June 1988; Flanagan, "Equality Rights."

77 RCS, *AIDS*; panel discussions at National Conference on AIDS, May 1988; "AIDS Fight: Should Junkies Get Free Needles?" *TS*, 3 July 1988; "Syringes Given to Drug Addicts in AIDS Fight," *TS*, 13 Oct. 1988; "Some MDs Giving Needles to Addicts to Combat AIDS," *TS*, 15 Oct. 1988; "Toronto Drug Users to Get Free Needles," *TS*, 13 Jan. 1989; "Ottawa Proposes Free Needles for Addicts," *TS*, 5 July 1989.

78 NAC RG 9, ser III B2, file 25–11–1 (1–8). Cassel, *Secret Plague*, chap. 6.

79 NAC RG 24, boxes 6617–8, files HQ 8994–6; HQC 8994–12, reel C 5318; HQC 60–4–19, reels C 5048–9; and RG 29, box 494, file 311–V3–29(3–5). Many pamphlets and lectures are in NAC RG 29, boxes 208–210, file 311–V3–3. See also Feasby, *Official History*, vol. 2, chap. 7, and Pierson, "Double Bind."

80 Tice et al., "Sources and Modes" and "Some Observations."

81 Copy of pamphlet in NAC RG 29, box 208, file 311–V3–3(2), and RG 24, box 6618, file HQ 8994–6(11); portions are illustrated in Pierson, "Double Bind," 50; "He 'picked up' more than a girl," NAC photograph C-12777.

82 Tice et al., "Some Observations," 54.

83 Cassel, *Secret Plague*, chap. 9.

84 Health Reports of Canada and the provinces. Canada, Commons, *Debates* (1943), 3176–9, (1944), 3025–8, 3031–2; NAC RG 29, boxes 207–210, file 311–V3–3; box 215, file 311–V3–19; box 216, file 311–V3–20; boxes 219–220, file 311–V3–22 (parts 9–13); boxes 493–7, file 311–V3–29. Health League of Canada, VD files 1939–46, NAC MG 28, I 332. H. Groulx, "Considérations pratiques en marge de la loi pour prévenir les

maladies vénériennes," *UMC* 71 (1942): 729–33; G. Choquette et E. La-
lande, "La Lutte antivénérienne dans la province de Québec," *UMC* 72
(1943): 877–80; A. Groulx, "La Lutte contre les maladies vénériennes à
Montréal," *UMC* 73 (1944): 794–8; E. Lalande and J. Archambault,
"Administration of a Provincial Venereal Disease Control Program,"
CJPH 35 (1944): 55–9; C.A. Bourdon, "Contribution du Service de
Santé dans la lutte antivénérienne à Montréal," *UMC* 76 (1947): 470–5;
H.C. Rhodes and D.E.H. Cleveland, "Venereal Disease Education in
Industry," *CJPH* 34 (1943): 494–501; E. LePage, "The Fight against
Venereal Disease," *CN* 40 (1944): 407–9; P. Capelle, "The Nurse and
Venereal Disease Control," *CN* 40 (1944): 487–8; B.D.B. Layton,
"The Practising Physician and the Control of Syphilis," *CMAJ* 63
(1950): 436–40.

Examples of media coverage: "Can Reduce Venereal Diseases to
Vanishing Point," *GM*, 13 May 1943; "Toll of Venereal Diseases," *GM*,
28 June 1943; "Terrifying Magnitude of Venereal Diseases," *GM*,
7 Dec. 1943; "Says Hush-Hush Talk Hurts Disease Cure," *TS*, 7 Dec.
1943; "VD ... No. 1 Saboteur," *Maclean's*, 15 Feb. 1944; "This is What
VD Costs," *Maclean's*, 1 Nov. 1944; "Four Worthy Suggestions," *GM*,
6 Oct. 1944; "Venereal Disease: Amateur Carriers," *GM* 9 Nov. 1944;
"Eradicate VD Claxton Urges," *GM*, 8 Feb. 1945; "Could Eradicate
Syphilis in 10 Years," *GM*, 3 Dec. 1945; "Proper Education in Sex Is
Declaired Major VD Weapon," *GM*, 7 Feb. 1946; "Attack Social Dis-
eases," *TS*, 8 Dec. 1943; "Greatest Health Problem," *TS*, 25 Jan. 1944;
"Toronto Opens War on Social Diseases," *TS*, 15 May 1944; "The Next
Great Plague to Go," *TS*, 26 Oct. 1944; "Predicts Eradication of VD,"
TS, 13 Nov. 1944; "Urges Persistent Education To Fight Venereal Dis-
ease," *TS*, 12 Sept. 1945.

85 Health Reports for Canada and the provinces. Dominion Council of
Health Minutes, 1950–1962; NAC RG 29, boxes 1234–5, file 311–v3–1;
MG 28 I 332, VD files 1947–67; *Fifth Western Regional Conference of Direc-
tors of VD Control, Vancouver, February 1950*, p 57 (in NAC RG 29,
box 210); R. Miller, "The Facts of Life," *CMAJ* 94 (1966): 147; F.M.F.
Richards, "Sex Education in the Schools – The Doctor's Role," *CMAJ*
95 (1966): 924–6; A. McCreary-Juhasz, "Sex Knowledge of Prospective
Teachers and Graduate Nurses," *CN* 63 (1967): 48–50; G. Szasz, "Sex
Education and the Public Health Nurse," *CJPH* 60 (1969): 429–34.

86 Annual Health Reports; NAC RG 29, box 1235–6, file 311–v3–1 (3–7)
and file 311–v3–3; "Facts on VD Ignored," *GM*, 17 Aug. 1968; numerous articles in *GM* and *TS*, Apr.–June 1971; "Alberta Task Force Recommendations," *CMAJ* 115 (1976): 276–7; Manitoba Department of
Health, *Venereal Disease Public Awareness Campaign, 1978 Report*;
Meltzer, "STD in Canada"; W.W. Watters, J.A. Lamont, J. Askwith,

and M. Cohen, "Education for Sexuality: The Physician's Role," CFP 27 (1981): 1941–44; Sacks, Bowie, and Stayner, "Education and Public Awareness"; Adrien et Carsley, "Éléments d'un programme"; Rodway and Wright, *Decade of the Plague*.

87 L. Cohen, "Federal Centre"; "Ottawa Role in AIDS Fight Said 'Appalling,'" TS, 4 June 1987; "Will Ontario Meet Obligation in AIDS Fight?" TS, 29 Jan. 1988; "$7 million AIDS Campaign To Hit Every Ontario Household," TS, 22 Mar. 1988; "Calls Triple to AIDS Hotline after Start of Ad Campaign," TS, 9 Apr. 1988; RSC, *AIDS*; National AIDS Conference, 16–18 May 1988; "Canada's Fight against AIDS Failing Miserably," TS, 16 Apr. 1989.

88 Methods are recorded in material cited in nn 88–91.

89 "Venereal Disease Hotline Gives Round-the-Clock Information," CN 67, no. 12 (Dec. 1971): 15.

90 On problems, see material in nn 83–6.

91 "Here's What Was Said on Talk CBC Censored," TS, 15 Jan. 1963.

92 In addition to sources in n 87, see, e.g., "Bus Shelter Posters to Launch AIDS Education Campaign," TS, 5 June 1987; "Ontario Fairs to Offer AIDS Details," TS , 31 Aug. 1987. Copies of pamphlets and posters are held by CGA, CAS, ACT, and ministries of health.

93 J.M. Last, "Ethics, Mores and Values – and AIDS," CJPH 78 (1987): 75–6; "Critics Attack TV Group for Rejecting AIDS Ads" and "Canadian AIDS Ad Judged Worst," TS, 27 Mar. 1987; "Tough Measures on AIDS Needed Broadcasters Say," TS, 18 Apr. 1987; "Broadcasters Plan Attack on AIDS," TS, 30 Sept. 1987; "AIDS Ads Can Offend: Broadcaster," TS, 16 Nov. 1987; "AIDS Ad Blitz Hits Roadblock," TS, 23 Mar. 1988; "TV Networks Deny Rejecting AIDS Ads," TS, 9 June 1989.

94 Ontario, *AIDS Let's Talk*; "Lifesaving Words: Ontarians Getting Facts on AIDS," TS, 23 Mar. 1988.

95 "Fighting a Tide of Ignorance," TS, 14 Dec. 1985; "A Day ont he AIDS Hotline," TS, 11 Feb. 1986; "Drive Planned to Stop Spread of Deadly AIDS," TS, 5 June 1986; "A Campaign To Promote Safe Sexual Practices in the Montreal Homosexual Population," CDWR, 13/3, 24 Jan. 1987; "Program To 'Eroticize' Safe Sex Being Planned," TS, 23 Mar. 1987; "Frank Talk in War on AIDS," TS, 11 Jan. 1989; RSC, *AIDS*; National AIDS Conference, 16–18 May 1988; "Take It Off, Put It On," ACT poster, Apr. 1988; ACT pamphlets: *Oral Sex*, Oct. 1988, *Anal Sex*, Jan. 1989, CGA ACT Archives.

96 See nn 83–5.

97 This observation is made by Pierson, "Double Bind," 46.

98 See n 86. Copies of pamphlets are preserved in NAC RG 29 and MG 28 I 332. The classic pamphlet from the 1970s and 1980s is Canada, NHW, *Sexually Transmitted Diseases*.

99 A.D. Bowd, "Knowledge and Opinions about AIDS among Student Teachers and Experienced Teachers," *CJPH* 78 (1987): 84–7; "Fear and Ignorance on AIDS Widespread in Canada," *TS*, 14 Dec. 1987; "The AIDS Message Is Not Getting Through," *TS*, 15 Dec. 1987; C. Gray, "Myths about AIDS Continue To Flourish," *CMAJ* 138 (1988): 733–4; National Conference on AIDS, May 1988; "Heterosexuals and AIDS," *TS*, 30 July 1988; "AIDS Survy Aims to Target Education Where It's Needed," *TS*, 5 Feb. 1989; "La Crainte du sida n'a pas modifié le comportement sexuel des Québécois," *PR*, 3 June 1989.

100 See, e.g., M.L. Foster, "Sex Education? By Whom?" *CPHJ* 9 (1918): 229–30; M. Patterson, "What To Teach about Parenthood and How To Teach It," *CPHJ* 10 (1919): 523–5; P. Sandiford, "The School Programme and Sex Education," *CPHJ* 13 (1922): 59–62; J.J. Heagerty, "Relative Value of Sex Education," *CPHJ* 15 (1924): 258–61. Vancouver City Health Department, ser. 1, box 103 B1, file "Health Education in Schools 1910–1925" contains correspondence from across Canada on arrangements for sex education. G. Desjardins, "La Pédagogie du sexe: un aspect du discours catholique sur la sexualité au Québec 1930–60," *Revue d'histoire de l'Amérique française* 43 (1990): 381–401.

101 H.C. Rhodes and D.E.H. Cleveland, "Venereal Disease Education in the High School," *CJPH* 35 (1944): 182–9; "A Challenge to the Schools," *TS*, 29 Nov. 1944; Dominion Council of Health Minutes, 47th meeting, 28–9 May 1945, 48th meeting, No.–Dec. 1945; Canada, Commons, *Debates*, 29 Mar. 1945; *Report of Venereal Disease Commission, Manitoba, 1946*, 28–9; Departement of Pensions and National Health, "A Manual of Educational Techniques in Venereal Disease Control," 1945, NAC RG 29, box 208, file 311–V3–3(4); "VD as Isolated Subject in Schools Held Wrong," *GM*, 6 Nov. 1948.

102 G. Desjardins, "La Pédagogie du sexe: un aspect du discours catholique sur la sexualité au Québec 1930–60," *Revue d'histoire de l'Amérique française* 43 (1990): 381–401; "School Sex Education Urged To Combat VD," *TS*, 4 Mar. 1965; R. Miller, "The Facts of Life," *CMAJ* 94 (1966): 147; F.M.F. Richards, "Sex Education in the Schools – The Doctor's Role," *CMAJ* 95 (1966): 924–6; A. McCreary-Juhasz, "Sex Knowledge of Prospective Teachers and Graduate Nurses," *CN* 63 (1967): 48–50; L.L. Keyes and H.M. Parrish, "Increasing the Effectiveness of Venereal Disease Education," *CJPH* 59 (1968): 119–22; "Schools To Be Encouraged To Offer Instruction on VD," *GM*, 14 May 1969; R.M.F. Manual and R.L. Persad, "Venereal Disease Education Using a Teaching Questionnaire," *CJPH* 62 (1971): 336–9; A.V. Vandermaas, "Integrated Sex Education," *CFP* 20 (1974): 94–6; D.B. Ulis, "Vie familiale et éducation sexuelle au Canada: une vue d'ensemble," *CJPH* 66 (1975): 114–21; "Alberta Task Force Recommendations,"

CMAJ 115 (1976): 276–7; W.W. Watters et al., "Education for Sexuality: The Physician's Role," *CFP* 27 (1981): 1941–4; S.L. Sacks et al., "Education and Public Awareness of Sexually Transmitted Diseases," *CJPH* 74 (1983): 176–8; J. Savage, "How Physicians Can Introduce Sex Education in Schools," *CFP* 31 (1985): 789–91; B.L. Cull-Wilby et al., "The Relationship between Sex Education and Knowledge in Grade Eight Students," *CJPH* 76 (1985): 163–6; A. King, "Education Research," National AIDS Conference, Toronto, 16 May 1988; "Author Gives Sex Education a Failing Grade," *TS*, 23 June 1989.

103 Bowd, "Knowledge among Teachers"; "Vander Zalm Upset over Methods Used To Warn about AIDS," *TS*, 30 Apr. 1987; "No Sex' Plea Won't Help AIDS Fight," *TS*, 15 May 1987; "Ontario To Teach Grade 7 Students about AIDS Danger," *TS*, 10 June 1987; "Catholic Schools AIDS Project Gets Approval," *TS*, 16 Oct. 1987; National Conference on AIDS, May 1988, espec. A. King, "Education Research"; "Teenagers Well-Versed on AIDS Nation-Wide Youth Survey Finds," *TS*, 17 May 1988; "Majority Want School Courses To Stress Importance of Sale Sex," *TS*, 13 June 1988; "Teens Fear AIDS but Don't Use Condoms, Study Shows," *GM*, 22 Oct. 1988; "Students Who Take AIDS Class Better Informed, Study Finds," *TS*, 28 Jan. 1989; "Manitoba Education Criticized by Study," *TS*, 31 Mar. 1989; "Straight Talk on AIDS, the New Facts of Life," *CPHA* video, released June 1989; "L'école pourrait faire mieux," *PR*, 3 June 1989; "Sex Disease Epidemic Feared as Students Ignore Condoms," *TS*, 20 June 1990.

Equity and Health Care

ROBIN F. BADGLEY AND
SAMUEL WOLFE

As part of the milestone social-security measures enacted by Parliament in 1966, the objectives set for the Medical Care Bill were to eliminate economic barriers in access to insured medical services and remove regional disparities in the provision of these services. The bill's companion pieces tabled by the minority Liberal government were the Canada Assistance Plan, a 40 per cent increase in benefits under the Guaranteed Income Supplement for the Aged, and the Health Resources Fund bill, providing for an expansion of training resources for heath-sciences personnel and the construction of new hospitals and laboratories. Together with other measures, the ultimate goal of this legislative package was "the elimination of poverty among our people."[1]

The Medical Care Act came into force on 1 July 1968. Since then, access to medical care has become accepted as an entrenched right in this country. Speaking to an American audience in 1987, Marc Lalonde, who had been minister of Health between 1972 and 1977, observed that "of all the public programs in Canada, our public health insurance system ... has been consistently the most popular since its creation. No one political party in Canada is suggesting fundamental changes to it."[2]

Despite being widely accepted as a success story at home and abroad,[3] no consolidated review of national health insurance has ever been undertaken by government to assess directly the extent and nature of class differences in health status and access to health care. This lack of official interest contrasts with the widely known findings of the 1980 Black Report for Great Britain and the recommendations of several Canadian advisory reports (Epp, Evans, Podborski, and Spasoff) that reducing social inequities in health must be priorities for social policy.[4] For its part, the research community has done little to fill this void. The few reviews undertaken lack a historical perspective, uncritically accept reported findings, and draw upon available Canadian research documentation selectively.[5] For these reasons, little is known about the major beneficiaries of national health insurance and particularly whether the access to care and the health of those previously known to be at high risk in terms of illness – the poor, the disabled, and the unemployed – have improved.

Beyond occasional legislative rhetoric, the official lid on this Pandora's box remains tightly closed, limiting the opportunity for broader public consideration. This general lack of attention to the issue of class and health also stems in part from the widely held belief that Canada has become a more egalitarian society in recent years. While this comfortable idea is unsupported in terms of there having been any appreciable income redistribution between rich and poor,[6] it is assumed that the social quality of life has kept pace with the country's overall high standard of living, and the plight of those in need had been considerably relieved by the broad blanket of welfare reforms established since the Second World War.

For the most part recent social-policy initiatives taken by government have focused upon cost containment and ensuring equality of opportunity in access to benefits rather than seeking to alter those features of the social system that serve to perpetuate engrained inequality. Inherent in this perspective is the idea that if services are accessible to all, then each has an equal chance and responsibility to achieve parity. T.H. Marshall has observed of the British health system that this attitude not only tends "to make poverty invisible; it also inhibits recognition of the many features of the social system which prevent equal opportunity from becoming a fact – as well as an ideal, and encourages the belief that individual failure, and poverty in general, are primarily a result of personal shortcomings."[7]

As voiced by Monique Begin, minister of Health and Welfare 1977–84, and subsequently echoed by her successors from 1986 to 1989,[8] this complacent perspective discourages policy attention from focusing directly upon class divisions in health care. In *Medicare: Canada's Right to Health*, published in 1987, the former minister reiterated the view held by many others that "our health care system is one of the best in the world, perhaps the best from any point of view you want to use: efficiency, cost, quality, distribution … Everyone has equal access to quality health care."[9]

How valid are such assertions? Do all have equal access? If they do, are the poor any better off than before? In seeking answers to these questions, this review draws upon the historical research record dealing with class divisions and health in Canada. Among the several different meanings in common usage attributed to the concepts of equality and equity, three dimensions are considered here. Is there reasonable access to uniform benefits provided on a basis to meet variable individual needs? Have gaps in health status between the poor and other Canadians narrowed as a result of social-security programs, including national health insurance? And is there reasonable equality of participation in establishing priorities where the concerns of a population are paramount, not those of special groups or classes?

THE GREAT FORWARD STEP

Building upon a foundation of federal and provincial initiatives spanning several decades, the Medical Care Bill tabled on 12 July 1966 was hailed by its legislative pilot as "going a long way toward closing the gap in our over-all social security system." The coverage then available to the population of about twenty million persons, Allan J. MacEachen reported, was that "some 6 million Canadians still lack any medical insurance coverage, and 3 million more have only limited coverage. Probably not more than 10 million Canadians at the present time have what would be called adequate comprehensive coverage. Those without adequate coverage include primarily residents of rural areas and people with moderate or low incomes."[10]

The main conditions set out in Bill C-227 were to assure universal coverage for medically insured services, portability of benefits, and a co-financed program administered by the provinces. These administrative features were based upon several overarching principles, some embodying conflicting purposes for achieving equity in health care. Now forgotten in some quarters and qualified by hindsight in others, the achieving of greater equity in health and in access to health care were foremost among these policy goals.

Marking "an historic day for this parliament," the government, in the minister's words, recognized "the fundamental principle that health is not a privilege but rather a basic right which should be open to all." In addition to this humanitarian concern, the state of the people's health was seen as a barometer of the country's social and economic development. The attainment of good health "is of direct benefit to the wider community"; the nation cannot "afford the loss to our economy stemming from ill health".

The new health policy focused upon eliminating two invidious economic barriers. At the individual level, "the opportunity for good health ... should be available to every citizen of our country ... irrespective of their ability to pay." While not defined, access to care was to be provided on a "reasonable" basis. To avert the levying of user charges and medical extra-billing, the bill further specified that federal payments could be withheld to the extent that this occurred.

The second barrier to be removed was the phasing out of regional economic disparities in the provision of medical services. Recognizing that "not all of the provinces have the same fiscal capability of providing ... programs designed for all residents," the plan would "ensure ... establishing an acceptable level of services available to all citizens." With Ottawa paying half of the costs calculated on a combined national coverage, this arrangement was geared to assist those provinces below this level, particularly the Maritimes. It was this group, the minister noted, that was "less capable financially of bearing the burden of a medical care program. We thought this was a fair procedure."[11]

Like the 1942 Beveridge Report for Great Britain, the 1964 Hall Report, upon which the government's new bill was based, forecast that the introduction of national health insurance in Canada would result in an initial rise in expenditures followed by a levelling off as unmet needs were provided for.[12] While NDP members in Parliament endorsed the view that there would be a redistribution but not a continuing increase in costs, the government benches remained silent on this issue. In the early 1960s national health expenditures were above 5 per cent of the gross national product (GNP); by 1989 this share had grown to 8.9 per cent.[13] Compared to other Western industrialized nations, during this period Canada developed and has continued to maintain a relatively plump health-care system. In 1983, it ranked fourth in terms of per capita health expenditures, and then moved to between second and third place globally during the remainder of the 1980s.[14]

During C-227's Bill third reading in 1966, Mitchell Sharp, minister of Finance, forecast that costs would grow for the first five years while provincial plans were being established. To foster the consolidation of this important "nation-wide advance," the open-ended co-financing agreement with the provinces would be retained during this period of development. These terms would then be renegotiated under a tax-equalization formula for established programs providing the provinces with greater budgetary autonomy. This anticipated realignment (effected later under the Established Programs Financing Act of 1977) would no longer tie Ottawa's contribution directly to program costs and preclude the federal auditing of provincial accounts.[15]

Prior to its tabling, T.C. Douglas, the pioneer of pace-setting health reforms in Saskatchewan, had forecast that the passage of this legislation would be "one of the great steps forward in the social history of Canada."[16] There was strong agreement in Parliament that this was "an idea whose time had come." Although the measure was broadly supported, the questions of eliminating class inequalities in health and access to care were minor items for discussion on the political agenda. Of seventy-eight speakers debating this bill, only one in six referred directly to the issue of poverty and illness. Most of the comments here were trivial asides or little more than political posturing – as, for instance, opposition to the postponement of the initially announced starting date by a year to 1 July 1968. In addition to the minister of Health, only three other members of Parliament (T.C. Douglas, David Lewis, and John Munro) spoke in depth and with compassion about health care as a basic right, the hoped for redistributive benefits of the plan, and the need to rub out the indignity and humiliation of being subjected to economic means tests before receiving needed services.

Reflecting concerns that were to dominate legislative attention in the years following its passage, most of the debate of Bill C-227 focused upon preserving or extending the powers of the private sector and professional interests. Instead of a publicly administered plan, the official opposition called for broadening the scope of voluntary health insurance operated by the private sector. Several members of Parliament who were physicians sought assurances that the traditional autonomy of the medical profession would not be jeopardized by state medicine. Both opposition parties demanded a widening of the definition of "unsured medical" services. The justification offered was less to expand services needed by the population than to ensure that the rights and opportunities of excluded health occupations, such as chiropractors, would not be eroded. The acceptance of this amendment for those provinces choosing to share broader co-financed expenditures assured that the range of services available would not be uniformly offered across the country.

How greater equity in health care was to be achieved rested upon several policy assumptions underlying this legislation and in the administrative conditions enacted. Foremost among these was the belief that the operation of a single program by itself could alter or eliminate problems of access at both individual and structural levels.

In establishing the principle of equality of access, the intent was that class divisions in obtaining care would disappear, with need becoming the main criterion for seeking medical treatment. Once the economic barrier was removed, it was expected that the health of all Canadians would improve, particularly among low-income groups.

The idea of demand then in vogue was one-sided, the presumption being that there was a relatively fixed relationship between the supply of personnel and the use of their services, the latter being largely a function of meeting patients' needs. Beyond an initial expansion as the national program became established, no later sharp increase in the supply of health manpower was anticipated, nor was it expected that there would be any significant change in the workstyle, organization, or payment of medical practice, then provided largely on a fee-for-service basis.

At the level of the organization of medical care, uniform services of high quality were to be established across Canada. This structure was to evolve within a range of provincially defined "insured" services, others included by the provinces on an optional basis and in the absence of central monitoring mechanisms assessing the quality of performance. Notably, none of the plan's five basic conditions was operationally defined. Also, in conjunction with the provision of the Health Resources Fund Act of 1966, it was expected that there would be a gradual levelling-out through time in the distribution of health facilities and personnel across the country.

The Medical Care Bill was passed by a vote of 177 to 2 on 8 December 1966. Three years after its terms came into force on 1 July 1968, all provinces and the two territories had joined the plan. Since then, while its financing formula was later renegotiated and its administrative conditions more clearly defined, the plan's basic features have remained intact. The Established Programs Financing Act of 1977 transferred tax points to the provinces combined with a direct federal contribution indexed to changes in the nation's GNP. This new block-funding arrangement provided the provinces with greater autonomy in the operation of their health plans and largely eliminated federal fiscal monitoring of the provincial plans.

During the first four years following the acceptance of the 1977 revision, the provinces gained some $666 million more than they would have received under the initial provisions. As well, additional sources of revenue came from user charges for certain hospital services and extra-billing fees collected by some physicians above provincially set payment rates. Only the residents of three eastern provinces were exempt from these practices.[17] In Alberta these levies were assessed on many who were social-assistance recipients, the elderly and the working poor.[18] Despite being opposed by the provinces and rejected by the president of the Canadian Medical Association as "constitutional rape,"[19] the Canada Health Act of 1984 was unanimously passed by Parliament in order to eliminate these economic barriers at the level of direct patient care. During the first nine months of the application of this legislation, some $86 million in federal sanctions were invoked against provinces continuing to permit the collection of additional charges.[20]

Although all provinces subsequently confirmed the act's terms, there were still abundant signs that official sanctions had not precluded substantial variation in extra health costs being directly paid by patients, nor had sophisticated billing practices been eliminated for services not covered in the provincial plans. Reacting to the new billing restrictions, a growing number of physicians began to develop annual fee plans exempting patients from paying for uninsured services.[21] In some instances, the cost ranged from $40 for individuals to $70 for families. Non-subscribers were billed for uninsured services, such as $7.50 for telephone advice, $20 for missed appointments, and $50 for special physical examinations. Another by-product of the ban on extra-billing charges may have been its impact in fostering the submission of both more expensive and a larger number of claims to provincial health plans. In Ontario such billings rose annually by 2 per cent during the years following the act's passage in 1984.[22]

REGIONAL DISPARITIES

Historically there have been sharp regional disparities in aggregate wealth and standards of living across Canada. While there has been some shuffling of positions, in general an east-to-west gradient still persists, with the eastern provinces ranking the lowest on a range of economic indicators. With respect to average personal income, the disparity gap (ratio of highest to lowest) between the provinces was 2.03 in 1961 and 1.69 in 1981.[23] During this period the unemployment gap was 4.75 in 1961 and 3.72 in 1981. In each instance the Maritimes trailed the rest of the country.

The often amended but continuing program of federal transfer payments was instituted to redress these durable regional disparities. The principle of promoting greater interprovincial equalization was also incorporated in other legislation, such as national health insurance. Under the federal Medical Care Act, higher equalization payments were initially made to the poorer provinces, a situation partly reversed following 1977, when taxation loopholes provided a fiscal dividend to the wealthiest provinces. This advantage was eliminated in 1982, when the method of calculating the federal contribution was revised so that all provinces were then receiving approximately comparable support. In 1986, in order to reduce the federal debt, provincial equalization payments have been incrementally scaled down, a shift that has resulted in a higher proportion of provincial budgets being allocated for health expenditures.

National health insurance provided an essential threshold of benefits for all Canadians. In relation to the distribution of physicians and hospital beds, there was a substantial levelling-out of long-standing regional disparities. By the mid-1980s there was no consistent variation in terms of the regional distribution of these services across the country, although substantial high-low gaps remained.[24] Transcending the benefits provided under the national plan, however, the aggregate wealth of a province or region still had a profound impact upon the scope and types of health care available to residents. People living in poorer regions still paid more from provincial tax funds for basic insured services, spent substantially less on health care for each individual, and received a narrower range of certain services, those relying upon new medical technology in particular.

In comparison with the wealthier western provinces, the eastern third of the nation assigned almost double the proportion of its regional gross domestic product on insured health service in 1978–79.[25] Alberta spent 3.9 per cent of its GDP on these services and Saskatchewan 5.1 per cent; in contrast, Newfoundland and Prince Edward Island respectively spent 8.9 and 9.4 per cent. In 1980–81 federal per capita transfers to the provinces ranged from $541 for Alberta to $1,298 for Prince Edward Island. In turn this federal support constituted 12 per cent of Alberta's provincial revenues and 56 per cent of those for Prince Edward Island. For the Maritimes as a whole, federal transfers accounted for more than half of provincial revenues. In terms of the amount spent on health care for each individual in 1985–86, this east-to-west pattern remained, with the four western provinces spending 18.9 per cent more than the four eastern provinces ($993.23 compared to $1,181.01).[26]

Whether there have been "spectacular gains"[27] or a widening of provincial differences in the supply of health resources through time depends upon which source of information is drawn upon and how findings are grouped. For the period between 1975–76 and 1985–86, federal reports indicate that the high-low gap in per capita health spending across the provinces rose from 31 per cent to 41 per cent.[28]

This trend is reflected in the provincial distribution of physicians. In 1964 the Royal Commission on Health Services forecast a manpower deficit by 1971.[29] This fear was unfounded. In 1961 the national doctor-to-population ratio was 1:857. By 1971 the ratio of 1:661 had surpassed the commission's estimates for 1991, and by 1990 this ratio had dropped to a national average of 1:518.[30] Although during these years the east-to-west gap in the distribution of physicians disappeared,[31] disparities remained between some of the poorer provinces and the more affluent. In 1961 British Columbia's physician-to-population ratio was 1:758, and this was reduced to 1:467 by 1986. In contrast, while less-well-off New Brunswick's ratio dropped from 1:1,314 to 1:764 during this period, the proportional gap between the two provinces had slightly widened.

If we look beyond the distribution of health personnel and hospital beds to how specific services are used, several measures indicate that the relative strength of a region's economy may influence the provision of assistance benefits and the extent to which specialized services are performed. With respect to social-welfare benefits, an east-to-west pattern occurs in the average amount of welfare support available to single disabled persons, lone-parent families, and employable individuals.[32] When the occurrence of five specialized surgical procedures is considered relative to provincial per capita income levels, a comparable trend emerges (see table on page 202). The rates per 100,000 for these procedures are drawn from 1984–85 national statistics and are grouped for each of the four provinces respectively having the lowest and highest average per capita incomes in 1986.[33] A similar but less marked interprovincial trend occurs for patients undergoing renal dialysis across Canada (Maritimes, 13.8/100,000; British Columbia, 19.7/100,000 in 1984).[34]

Citing the experience of Prince Edward Island, a task force appointed by the Canadian Medical Association concluded in 1984 that the uneven availability of new medical technology posed ethical and logistical dilemmas. "Medical situations may arise that dictate the need for immediately available facilities ... the lack of technology ... also results in a failure to attract specialists to the region."[35]

Specialized medical services also continued to be unevenly distributed within provinces, making their accessibility partially a function of where a person lived. In 1987 six of ten medical centres providing the amniocentesis procedure in Ontario were university-affiliated teaching hospitals. Four hospitals accounted for 89.4 per cent of the procedures performed.[36] An earlier review of genetic diagnostic services for Manitoba found that "although 60 per cent of the women of that province over age 35 live outside of Winnipeg, 85 per cent of referrals were from Winnipeg and only 15 per cent from other parts of Manitoba." Part of a broader review of genetic

Surgical Procedures by Provincial per capita Income 1986

Surgical procedures (1984–85)	Four lowest provinces	Four highest provinces (rate per 100,000)	National average
computer axial tomography	59.6	102.7	93.5
diagnostic ultrasound	97.4	180.7	166.0
bypass heart revascularization	28.7	33.5	32.8
hip replacement/ arthroplasty	59.5	105.8	58.9
knee-ankle arthroplasty	28.3	37.6	36.2

programs in Montreal, Toronto, and Vancouver, the Winnipeg report also cited "unanimous concern ... that the greater the income and education, the more likely the woman is to seek prenatal diagnosis."[37]

When we draw together the trends in the distribution of health resources across Canada, it becomes apparent that substantial gains have been made in the levelling-out of the provision of front-line services. Complementing this shift, outcome measures such as infant-mortality rates and longevity have also become regionally more uniform than in the past. Despite these gains, other disparities remain, including differential spending per capita on health care and the availability of some medical services. While the documentation here is incomplete and needs to be augmented, available evidence indicates that a region's relative wealth serves to perpetuate differential access by individuals, particularly to highly specialized services located in tertiary-level-care urban hospitals. Under the revised federal-provincial health co-financing formulas between 1982 and 1992 and the retrenchment of regional programs announced in the 1989 federal budget, indications are that the disparities noted will remain and may become wider in the years ahead.

ACCESS TO MEDICAL CARE

During the past half-century several dozen studies have focused upon the social and economic backgrounds of individuals relative to their use of health services. In addition to providing a baseline to assess changes that evolved later, the studies conducted prior to the introduction of national health insurance identify broader dimensions of health care that have often been ignored by later investigators. In most of the earlier studies there was a clear recognition of the concept of poverty, the effect of social class on access to care and ill health, and the identification of high-risk groups such as the unemployed, the disabled, and poor children. In contrast, most of the recent utilization studies have ignored these vital concerns. Their narrow focus upon the use of hospital and medical services alone precludes an assessment of the appropriateness of the care provided in relation to the needs of patients.

Studies before National Health Insurance

The first major Canadian analysis of class and health was conducted by economist Leonard Marsh and two medical colleagues in Montreal during the Depression of the 1930s. Marsh was then on short-term appointment as the director of Research in the Social Sciences at McGill University. In his training at the University of London he had participated in studies led by Sir William Beveridge. Drawing upon the findings of six surveys focusing mainly upon the experience of some 4,600 unemployed and employed blue-collar workers, the 1938 study documented occupational mortality rates, medical, hospital, and dental care, physical disabilities, and the height, weight, and nutritional status of children. Relying upon a breadth and detail of documentation seldom replicated since, Marsh and his colleagues concluded that "if medical care is a contingency left to each individual to secure as best he can, it becomes a function of the distribution of wealth." To break this ironclad relationship, they called for a program of comprehensive social security, including health-insurance benefits. With respect to the latter, this interdisciplinary research team cautioned that "the availability of medical attention when the emergency arises, however, is only part of the problem ... other conditions predisposing to sickness are themselves products of the subsistence level. Preventive treatment here must start at a stage further back with improved diets, better housing ... rather than the 'ambulance work' of medicine alone."[38] Thirty-seven years later Marsh reiterated that "in every civilized country, no social service is more basic than that of health care ... (yet) ... it is sad that the record reveals every variety of compromise and resistance."[39] He was personally well versed in the difficulties of changing traditional values. Despite the highly productive research program he directed from 1930 to 1940, Marsh's contract with McGill University was not extended because his collectivist philosophy and membership in the League for Social Reconstruction embarrassed a conservative academic administration.[40]

Between 1937 and 1939 an analysis funded by the Rockefeller Foundation compared the use of health services in Glace Bay and Yarmouth in Nova Scotia. Breaking new ground in Canadian health-care studies, the results showed that people in the community where doctors were paid in part by salary and workers had insurance coverage were not as sick but made more use of services than residents having no insurance scheme and living where doctors were paid fees. The study's main conclusion was that "the existence of an insurance plan will not only remove the economic barrier between doctor and patient, but will also have a profound influence on the patient's concept of the need for medical services ... [and the extension of benefits would] ... bring about a considerable rise in the demand for health services."[41]

After the Second World War Ottawa's attempt to introduce a comprehensive program of social security was thwarted because no agreement could be reached with the provinces, but starting in 1948 a program of national health grants was phased in supporting hospital construction, provincial public-health services, and research. As part of this initiative the Canadian Sickness Survey undertook a comprehensive appraisal of the health of some 36,000 Canadians in 1950–51. The information obtained drew upon interviews, health diaries, monthly visits, and verification of self-reports with medical charts.

Providing an important benchmark for comparison with later national surveys, this survey found no differences by income in the number of illnesses reported (about two each year) and hospital admissions (about one in ten hospitalized annually). There was a direct relationship with income, however, with respect to visits to doctors, surgical operations, all types of health care, and health expenditures. On average, 61.1 per cent having high incomes received some form of health care annually, compared to 45.3 per cent in the lowest income group. The former annually spent $158.70 on health care, in contrast to $46.60 by the latter. A strong inverse relationship with income occurred in terms of the amount of disability reported. The survey concluded that "ill health amongst persons in the low income group is more serious than amongst those with a medium or high income ... [and] ... the low income group had the smallest proportion of persons reporting care, except in the case of in-patient hospital care and home nursing services."[42] Standardized for age and sex, the average number of disability days each year was 17.8 for low-income persons and 9.6 for the high-income group.

The Canadian Sickness Survey noted that "the different pattern of disabling illnesses ... explains much of the relatively high amount of hospital care received by persons in the low income group" and that in this respect "the low income group appeared to be reasonably well served." The group "furthest behind" in receiving health care were the children of low-income families, while those "least far behind" were persons over sixty-five in the low-income group, many of whom received public assistance. As well, "for persons over 65, it was often the medium income group which received the least health care."[43]

The conclusions of these three early reports were in general confirmed and expanded upon by six later studies completed before the introduction of national health insurance.[44] One of these, the comprehensive study by the Leightons of psychiatric disorders in Stirling County (Digby), Nova Scotia, documented how the general disintegration of social bonds in the community was related to economic situation, the frequency of broken homes, and the rate of mental illness. Those in the lowest income group, many of whom were unemployed, had "a relatively high risk of psychiatric disorder, a high degree of impairment and large numbers of symptoms."[45]

The first before-and-after study of the impact of a public health-insurance plan was undertaken during the 1960s in a small prairie town in Saskatchewan.[46] That province had introduced a comprehensive program of hospital insurance in 1947. This was later followed by a provincial medical-care plan started in 1962 that sparked a bitter twenty-three-day doctors' strike. Two years before the plan came into effect a survey of the small community confirmed that the use of health services and the scope of insurance coverage varied by income. The second survey was conducted in 1965, three years after the introduction of the provincial plan. Although from 1960 to 1965 the use of medical services had narrowed between income groups, this had been accompanied by a realignment in how services were used, favouring those with higher incomes. The latter, in contrast to the less well off, were then making more use of non-insured services (for example, dental care) and a more sophisticated use of medically insured services (for example, seeking the care of urban specialists).

Prior to the introduction of national health insurance, the accumulated research evidence was reasonably firm and consistent in documenting sharp class divisions in the occurrence of illness, how services were used, and expenditures on health care. The needs of several high-risk groups were clearly identified – those living in poverty, particularly children, the unemployed, and the disabled. This early research relied upon a broad range of class measures and indicators of health status. The concept of health was comprehensive, encompassing the use of a range of services, the physical- and mental-health status of individuals, disability, and longevity. Some studies, notably those by Marsh and the Leightons, sought to identify the nature of the social and economic dimensions affecting health-care inequalities.

Following the introduction of national health insurance, well over two dozen Canadian studies have focused upon the use of health services by social class. About a third of these concluded that class differences had been eliminated, a quarter that the poor were using more services than before and also more than the rich, and the remainder that utilization was still directly a function of class position. If each of these later studies is assumed to be of equal weight and validity, then the composite evidence would appear to suggest that a notable policy achievement has been realized, with the national program contributing to a progressive redistribution by class in the use of health care. A closer examination of this body of evidence, however, leaves little room to be sanguine that the gains are substantial or genuine. In the main these studies are restricted to the analysis of a single service; many do not distinguish the nature, level, and quality of the care given, and in several instances the research design and methods used are seriously flawed.

Pro-Poor Outcome

Focusing upon the period immediately following the beginning of the new national program, seven of the nine studies citing a sharp rise in the use of services by the poor relied upon descriptive statistics in reaching this conclusion.[47] In four instances a misleading procedure was used of relying upon the combined rates for census or provincial averages as proxies to delineate individual variations by income level.

The study most widely cited as proof that the new national program had achieved its egalitarian intent is the 1969–72 before-and-after appraisal conducted in Montreal. Extensively reported in the medical literature,[48] these findings indicate that while the overall level of use of medical services had not risen during this period, medical visits by the lowest income group had increased from 6.6 to 7.8 per year, while those by higher-income earners fell slightly from 5.3 to 4.8. On the basis of the evidence given, these conclusions are at best tenuous.

A comparable before-and-after study conducted in the Eastern Townships of Quebec, a region stretching from the outskirts of Montreal to the American border, found no marked shift during this period in use of these services.[49] Drawing directly upon Quebec health-insurance records, a second survey between 1971 and 1975 of sixty-five medical-service areas across the province concluded that the "health insurance system does not appear to have effected a *relative* redistribution of medical services from high-income to low-income areas. It may have done so shortly after the introduction of Quebec Medicare, but since then the trend, if there is a real trend, has been more in the opposite direction."[50] Subsequent information drawing upon official Quebec medical-insurance records indicates that the average number of medical services received by all residents in Quebec rose by 17.8 per cent between 1970 and 1975.[51]

The contrasting observations in these studies about the experience of one province immediately following the introduction of the new program are accounted for by the different research methods and analytical procedures used. For instance, in its descriptive analysis of income relative to the use of medical services, the 1969–72 Montreal study did not use controls for family size, age, or ethnicity. Income categories were arbitrarily set, and visits to hospital and health-department clinics as well as to emergency rooms were excluded, sources of care known to be more extensively used by the poor.[52]

A research technique that introduces the problem of an ecological fallacy in the interpretation of findings was built into the design of four other studies reaching pro-poor conclusions.[53] This procedure involves, for instance, using the average income for census tracts or a province and imputing these combined rates to reflect the experience of all individuals within an area. Relying upon this approach, the 1974 Statistics Canada survey of 12,500 Canadians found that 69.4 per cent of persons earning less than $5,000 had consulted physicians during the previous year, compared to 65.7 per cent of those with incomes above $25,000. In terms of visits and their financial value, the study concluded that "low income families receive more than their share of benefits."[54] The reported medical expenditures cited in this survey were 30 per cent lower than those recorded by official sources, and denominators were not listed in the report's tables. In calculating health expenditures for income groups, this 1974 study combined household information with the average cost of a medical visit for the province where individuals lived, an extrapolation that ignored the nature of these visits, the gravity of illness, and the actual expenditures entailed. As other studies have shown, by just focusing upon visits without detailing their substance, this procedure, in addition to its other drawbacks, overestimates the benefits received by the poor and underestimates those actually received by other income groups.

No Relationship

In general, drawing upon the findings of larger and more representative surveys as well as more recently collected information, ten studies have concluded that relative parity by class has been achieved in the use of medical services.[55] In light of the extensive and consistent documentation in national health surveys that the poor experience more ill health and disability than other Canadians, these results suggest that their needs may be less well provided for in this regard. Five of these reports relied upon the powerful statistical techniques of multivariate analysis, an approach where several variables are considered together in seeking to explain variation in outcomes. In terms of its predictive utility, the use of this analytical approach in studies of the utilization of health services typically accounts for between 4 and 20 per cent of variance, meaning that a majority of the factors affecting why people may use these services cannot be explained. Frequently in these studies, insufficient attention is given to the classification of what is being reviewed; the issue of co-linearity is often ignored, and the social meaning of variables, such as health care or income, is inadvertently sanitized.

The first major study that found no relationship between class and the use of services was the International Collaborative Study on Medical Care Utilization, which obtained information in 1968 from 15,608 individuals in Saskatchewan, Alberta, and British Columbia.[56] Although Saskatchewan had then had its own provincial medicare program in operation for six years, no specific analysis documenting its impact was included in this important international research. Despite the study's initial finding that income was not related to the use of health services, a subsequent reanalysis of this information by R.D. Smith documented a relationship by class in terms of how preventive health and auxiliary services were obtained.[57]

In a little-known separate analysis, the World Health Organization International Collaborative Study linked household survey findings to official health-insurance records, a verification procedure initially used in the 1950–51 Canadian Sickness Survey and later by J. Siemiatycki in his 1974 Montreal survey. In the instance of hospital admission, a salient event not readily forgotten by most persons, there was 28 per cent over-reporting by low-income individuals, in contrast to 14 per cent in the highest income bracket.[58] In the 1974 Montreal study, under-reporting was respectively 28 and 25 per cent for low- and high-income groups.[59] To the extent that these seldom-replicated findings may occur more widely, they indicate that the reported utilization of medical and hospital services by the poor may be spuriously high.

For a reasonably accurate assessment to be made about how services are used, studies such as these indicate that a layered approach to research, involving self-reports and official records, should be adopted. Significantly, all of the mainstream recent reports that have drawn upon both sources of information or only on official records have confirmed the persistence of a positive relationship between social class and the use of health services.

Several national health surveys were conducted between 1978 and 1985, three of which did not collect information on the use of medical and hospital services.[60] The descriptive findings of one survey found no relationship by income and the use of medical services, while in another the pattern was comparable for all persons having between one and nine medical visits; beyond this level the poor received more services.[61] Only limited attention has been devoted in the main reports of these national surveys to income-related analysis. The classification of this measure has been inconsistent, lacked a clear rationale, and precluded an analysis of utilization and ill health relative to persons whose incomes are below the poverty line. The categories used here have grouped income by quintiles, regular intervals of $5,000, a mixture of $10,000 and $15,000 intervals, and Statistics Canada low-income cut-off levels for residents in cities of over 500,000 inhabitants. In the latter instance, this criterion was superimposed in the ranking of the income of all families surveyed, regardless of their residence across Canada. No common denominator was used; information on income was variously assembled for individuals, families, and households. With one exception – the 1985 Health Promotion Survey, which used metropolitan low-income cut-off levels – no allowance was made in the other surveys to control for income level by the number of persons in a family or household, or by community size and region.

A deep knowledge of social welfare or economics is not needed to recognize that unless family size is accounted for in such studies, there may be a blurring of class distinctions. In 1986, for instance, the poverty cut-off lines for Toronto were $10,668 for an individual and $21,708 for a family of four persons. In the absence of this distinction, the economic situation of a single middle-class person relative to the use of services is equated to that of a family of four living in poverty, and this bias is further compounded when the health experience of children is excluded.

The sampling framework of each of the recent national health surveys has contained a systematic class bias. The design of the 1978–79 Canada Health Survey, for example, which was also used in the other surveys, excluded persons living in the Yukon, Northwest Territories, other isolated regions, Indian reservations, and the homeless as well as those who were institutionalized, such as the mentally ill, the elderly, and patients in general hospitals. The exclusion of these groups, said to represent only 3 per cent of the population, effectively precludes consideration of many who may be at high risk in terms of their health and who are poor, and also introduces an income-levelling effect in the results obtained.

Using a multivariate statistical approach similar to that of several other studies, a reanalysis of the findings of the 1978–79 Canada Health Survey by a group of Ottawa investigators concluded that "the use or nonuse of services is unrelated to the economic status of the individual."[62] This study omitted the experience of a quarter (24.9 per cent) of the original survey. These were children under the age of 15, a group including high-risk poor children. For all non-responses, such as the 5.9 per cent whose income was unreported, the study assigned a value of zero rather than adopting the more valid procedure of deleting this group from the analysis. The economic status of individuals was ranked into non-specified income quartiles; no controls for income were used relative to family size or with respect to regional variations in the poverty line. At a national conference where the findings of the reanalysis were reviewed, the researchers acknowledged that "the r^2 values were very low, but what they were testing for was goodness of fit, using a logistic package."[63]

There can be little doubt that conclusions grounded upon analytical assumptions such as those noted in the reanalysis of the 1978–79 Canada Health Survey may on occasion be more an artefact of the research techniques used than a valid reflection of the actual experience of those being studied. It is hardly surprising that studies adopting this approach in the analysis of health-care utilization invariably account for so little of the variance, and hence conclude that there is no relationship between class and health care.

Pro-Rich Outcome

Between 1951 and 1990 Canada's income-security system only minimally altered income disparities between rich and poor. The total income of the top fifth of Canadian households was 42.8 per cent of the national total in 1951 and 42.1 per cent in 1990. For the lowest fifth this share was respectively 4.4 per cent in 1951 and 5.2 per cent in 1990. A 1986 review by the Canadian Council on Social Development showed that while until then the package of welfare measures had had a sharply progressive impact for those with low incomes, the cumulative support was regressive in its consequences for the lowest income group when considered within the broader context of benefits provided by state insurance programs and tax exemptions.[64]

While there has been no comparable review of the distribution of financial benefits by class for national health insurance, studies documenting a positive relationship between class and the use of health services have variously focused upon the financial value of the services received, extra-billing expenses, surgical operations and preventive health care, and the extent of illness and the use of services by the unemployed.[65] Four of these studies drawing directly upon official insurance records or medical files confirm the continued existence of inequalities proportional to those identified in the 1950–51 Canadian Sickness Survey. The most extensive of these reviews is the work of R.G. Beck and J.M. Horne covering the period 1963–75.[66] These researchers linked income-tax records with health-insurance files for the residents of Saskatchewan. The several reports by these two scholars document the gradient in the dollar value of the services received by income level, and they further show that when user fees were collected in that province between 1968 and 1971, it was the poor, the elderly, and those with larger families who were the most affected. Under a program of full insurance coverage in effect in 1967, persons with incomes less than $2,500 averaged $60.77 in medical and hospital benefits, in contrast to $117.99 for those whose incomes were above $15,000.

The 1978 Manga Report of Ontario's experience with health insurance combined the results of a provincial household survey with official health-insurance records.[67] As in the case of the Beck-Horne studies, there was a direct relation between the average health-insurance benefits received and income level, viz $159.31 ($0–3,999), $145.93 ($4,000–7,999), $202.07 ($8,000–13,999), $257.01 ($14,000–19,999), and $253.69 ($20,000 plus). Confirming the trends identified earlier in Wheatville, Saskatchewan, this report also found that higher income groups used more specialist and attendant services than other income groups, while the poor obtained a significantly higher share of their care at hospitals than the non-poor. A subsequent analysis conducted for the Ontario Council of Health linked Manga's household survey with Ontario health-insurance files and took into account whether physicians had "opted-in" or "out" of the medical-insurance program. This study found sharp and consistent differences between welfare recipients and the elderly in terms of their being at risk of extra-billing by physicians who had "opted out" of the program.[68]

While it dealt with only one procedure, the Report of the Committee on the Operation of the Abortion Law tabled in Parliament in 1977 revealed a not readily documented side of physician-patient financial transactions.[69] Among its extensive surveys this federal inquiry obtained information directly from 4,754 patients having legal abortions in eight provinces. One in five paid out-of-pocket medical charges, averaging $73.71. In some instances these charges amounted to several hundred dollars. In terms of their social backgrounds, a disproportionate number of the abortion patients who paid extra charges were young, less well educated, and foreign-born.

Beyond the coverage provided under national health insurance, which is augmented in some provinces by additional benefits, health-care costs also entail expenses for additional insurance costs, dental care, drugs, appliances, hidden extra-billing charges, and other services not covered by provincial programs. Added expenses, particularly affecting the poor and low-income earners, include the loss of hourly wages, transportation costs, and the provision of follow-up care. While this side of health care has received little research attention, a lack of evidence has not prevented some from making invalid assertions in this regard. A former federal deputy minister, for instance, declared at an international forum that following medicare there was "no direct financial burden on the patient, the only deterrents ... are the time and trouble involved."[70] With no supporting evidence, still others have asserted that "out-of-pocket expenses have been eliminated."[71]

Information on family expenditures collected by Statistics Canada in its periodic national surveys undercuts these claims. In 1964 high-income families spent 4.5 times more on health care than low-income families.[72] Following the introduction of national health insurance, while this disparity had narrowed, a substantial difference remained. In 1972 the rich still spent 3.3 times as much in direct out-of-pocket expenses as did the poor, and by 1982 this gap had regressed slightly to a ratio of 3.9. In nominal dollar values the spread was from $99 to $441 in 1964, from $106 to $455 in 1972, and from $241 to $953 in 1982. While these costs as a share of total family income declined overall during these two decades, the burden on the poor was consistently higher than that on the rich. The proportions were respectively 6.0 and 3.1 per cent in 1964, 2.8 and 2.3 per cent in 1972, and 2.5 and 2.1 per cent in 1982.[73]

Thus, in terms of both actual dollar value and as a share of total income, the rich continued to spend more than the poor on health care. The introduction of national health insurance did little to modify this regressive distribution. On the contrary, the benefits provided under this national program may have reinforced the disparity. By providing coverage for middle- and upper-income groups, a displacement effect appears to have occurred whereby these groups have been given the opportunity to purchase more health benefits and continue in this regard to outstrip the financial capability of the poor.

A repeated problem with the studies reviewed illustrates an important but seldom-raised issue of the effect of political philosophy inherent in the design of health-survey research. Since the close association between demographic and socio-economic variables is well known, this factor revolves about the sequential ordering of information in statistical analysis.

If social and economic variables, as is usually the case, are positioned as secondary or intervening variables, and this is coupled with imprecise definition and inadequate controls, then it is hardly surprising in light of their high degree of co-linearity with demographic characteristics that the explanatory power of these measures is minimal. For instance, the 1985 Royal Commission on the Economic Union reported that 58.6 per cent of the elderly live below the poverty line, with this rising to 65.6 per cent among elderly females. Of those who were poor, 62.9 per cent had only a primary-school education, and 41.9 per cent of single-parent families were in this income group.[74] Also, as noted, the use of income level in the absence of controls for family size or situation renders conclusions largely spurious relative to a poor-rich gradient. In this situation the more accurately and readily gauged demographic indicators, such as age and sex, assume priority, whereupon analysts may conclude that need rather than class affects health status or the use of services.

In contrast, if a powerful and distinctive criterion of social and economic opportunity such as unemployment, lone-parent families, and Indian/Inuit status or other sharply defined class measures are made the lead or primary variables for analysis, there emerges a targeted conceptual focus on the degree of association with health-service consumption. The review of the Canadian studies on the use of health services by social class also clearly underscores the need to develop more discrimininating measures of health-utilization outcomes. Merely gauging contacts with physicians by whether these occur or by the number of visits made tells us nothing about the dollar-value or quality of the care received, the variation in the selective use of services, the relationship of care to need, or whether the care provided is curative or preventive in nature.

Distributional Trends in Utilization

The central conclusion emerging from a review of the major studies on the utilization of health services undertaken following the introduction of national health insurance is that class inequalities still characterize the ways in which health care is obtained by Canadians. In terms of the research approaches used, the findings of many studies, particularly a high proportion of those reaching pro-poor or no-relationship conclusions, should be discounted. In some instances the statistical analysis was rudimentary, while in others insufficient controls were introduced that might have distinguished the effects of other variables influencing the use of services. Many of these studies relied upon simple and readily obtained service-utilization measures, such as visits to physicians, and ignored other relevant aspects of health care. Finally, most of these studies were single-point prevalence reviews lacking longitudinal baselines.

The evidence derived from official health-insurance records shows that most Canadians have made extensive use of hospital and medical-care benefits. The sizeable gain achieved by national health insurance was the provision of a common denominator of access to services for all Canadians. However, ensuring an equality of opportunity did not provide for an equality of accessibility in terms of the benefits received. While the amount of care rose for all persons, this gain did little to alter existing class differences in how patients obtained care or in how it was provided to them.

To have expected otherwise of a single measure, such as national health insurance, in the absence of broader structural changes in Canadian society would have been to impute reform capabilities that were not inherent in its legislative mandate. Other changes that have evolved since the introduction of national health insurance, such as the revised federal-provincial co-financing agreements between 1977 and 1992 and the evolution of cost-containment ceilings, have served to crystallize even further both regional economic differences and class-related disparities in accessibility to health care.

HEALTH STATUS AND LONGEVITY

The durable disparities in the provision and accessibility of health care are a function of the class structure of Canadian society, both in terms of direct consequences and indirectly, as class position affects the health status of individuals. It was in clear recognition of the need to redress these inequities that national health insurance was enacted. While not embodied in this legislation, one of its fundamental objectives was claimed to be a guarantee that "health is ... a basic right ... open to all."[75]

Well before the emergence of the national program, the 1950–51 Canadian Sickness Survey had documented that ill health and disability were more prevalent among the poor than among other groups in the population. This conclusion was buttressed by the research findings of the studies conducted during this period, virtually all of which drew upon information concerning health status.

Among the studies subsequently undertaken that focused upon the use of services, about half also documented selected dimensions of ill health. For the most part these findings are confirmed by the results of several recent national health surveys and numerous studies dealing directly with the relationship between class and health status (for example, work injuries and accidents, the emotional health of children of welfare families, ill health and stress among unemployed men and women, and nutritional and general health status).[76]

The same caveats noted previously in the interpretation of the findings of utilization studies also apply to reports dealing with the association between class and health status. Where, for instance, class measures were positioned as enabling or secondary variables, it was generally concluded that there was little or no relationship between these and their impact on health. A majority of these reports, however, found a positive relationship between the health of individuals and their class position, a conclusion also borne out by the results of the 1978–79 National Health Survey, the 1983–84 Canadian Health and Disability Survey, and the 1985 General Social Survey.

While findings on class and health in the 1978–79 survey have been only partially reported, the disparities cited are clear. *The Health of Canadians*, published in 1981, concluded that "indicators of social class such as education and income reflect important differences in health status, not merely in terms of overall prevalence of problems but, more importantly, with respect to the types of problems resulting in serious consequences. It is clear that people of lower-income groups and with lower levels of education do not enjoy the same level of health as those Canadians of higher social and economic status." In the survey's list of the prevalence of twenty-two categories of health problems by income quintiles, the lowest group ranked first in fifteen, high-income groups first in three, and there was no difference or an uneven distribution in four categories. Not only did the poor experience more ill health, but the problems faced were graver. Those with the highest prevalence among the rich were hay fever and allergies, skin disorders, and trauma. In contrast, the poor experienced double the rate of the rich for mental and sight disorders, anemia, and heart disease, and also higher levels for diabetes, hypertension, asthma, and dental problems. Good emotional health was also found to be related to "being in the mainstream of Canadian society, with a disproportionate number of the poor experiencing symptoms of anxiety, depression, and feelings of insecurity.[77]

Of the 126,698 individuals included in the 1983–84 Disability Survey, about one in eight (12.8 per cent) had some degree of disability.[78] Regressive gradients occurred with respect to their participation in the labour force, amount of education, and income level. Over two in three disabled persons (68.4 per cent) were not in the labour force, and the proportion having only a primary level of education was more than double that of other Canadians. Many of the disabled lived in poverty, with two-thirds having an income of less than $9,000 in 1983–84.

Focusing upon voluntary initiatives and self-help networks, the 1985 General Social Survey of 11,200 individuals collected information on self-rated health status and physical-activity limitations. Its results reconfirmed a strong negative association between social class and ill health. "Persons with activity limitation are more than twice as likely to come from households ... in the lowest income group ($15,000) as persons with no activity limitation (21% vs 9%)," and those "with more severe limitations are more likely to be older ... and ... in lower income households."[79]

The descriptive statistics on ill health and disability documented in these national surveys warrant fuller consideration and analysis relative to their important policy implications concerning the health status of the poor. Due to differences in research design and how key terms were defined, no direct comparison can be made between the results of these surveys and those of the 1950–51 Canadian Sickness Survey. In general, however, these were remarkably similar in documenting the continued greater occurrence of ill health and disability among the poor.

During the mid-1980s Canada ranked near the top of the countries of the world in terms of the average life expectancy of its people.[80] Life expectancy is a crude index of the social quality of life and the nature of health care. However, as a summary measure for comparing international experience of life-chances by social class, life expectancy, along with infant-mortality rates of specific groups, is the most significant gauge available of the overall health status of a population.

The major gains in life expectancy in Canada preceded the introduction of hospital insurance in 1958 and medical-care insurance in 1968. For instance, average life expectancy in Canada in 1926 was 58 years. This level rose successively to 61 years in 1931, 69 years in 1951, 70 years in 1956, and by 1989 to 73 years for men and 80 years for woman. These trends show that it has been factors other than national health insurance that have contributed to higher life expectancies for Canadians. As these levels rise, significant gains in average longevity become only marginally more feasible. The impact of providing even more in the way of health services, while crucial at the level of individual treatment, appears to have little aggregate impact or benefit in terms of extending longevity even further for a whole population.

Corroborating the findings of studies showing class differences in health and access to care are eleven reports completed between 1974 and 1983 documenting life expectancy by occupational background or income level. There is a broad consensus among these reports that the non-poor live longer than the poor, with R. Wilkins's widely cited work suggesting that this gap may have widened in recent years. At the ministerial level, these results have been acknowledged as "incontrovertible evidence" and as "the first challenge we face ... in reducing inequities."[81] However, with three exceptions, the problem of an ecological fallacy is incorporated in the design of the body of this research.[82]

In their 1974 report on social class and life chances, A. Billette and G.B. Hill drew on 2,265 case-controlled pairs of the deaths of males aged 25 to 64.[83] Representing a 15 per cent national sample, the cause of death, demographic information, and class position (gauged by the Blishen scale) were taken from information recorded on death certificates. Setting average life expectancy at 100, the lowest economic group was reported to have a relative mortality risk of 145, in contrast to 75 for the top category of workers. This 2:1 ratio was even higher for certain conditions, such as pneumonia or non-traffic accidents.

Except for a review of occupational mortality rates in British Columbia between 1950 and 1978,[84] and the 1990 report by Wolfson and co-authors which drew information from the Canada Pension Plan, each of the subsequent studies focusing upon longevity either relied upon census-tract averages in calculating differential mortality rates or developed an index combining weighted estimates from information about individuals and institutional averages. D.T. Wigle and Y. Mao's 1980 report analysed 81,465 deaths in 21 metropolitan census areas across Canada in 1971. The social-class ranking of decedents was calculated on the basis of the median household income of the census tract where they had lived, this statistic being combined with death and demographic information taken from death certificates. The major conclusion of these investigators was that "mortality rates .ɴ vary substantially by income level in Canada. Males in income groups 1 and 5, respectively, had life expectancies at birth of 72.5 and 66.3 years; the corresponding values for females were 77.5 nd 74.6 years."[85] While drawing only upon urban experience, this conclusion was generalized to all of Canada. Relying also upon census-tract median-household income levels, small studies reaching similar conclusions were conducted in Montreal in 1976 and 1981 and in Toronto between 1979 and 1985.[86]

The index of a population's health developed by Wilkins and Adams drew upon information from the 1978–79 Canada Health Survey, national hospital statistics, 1970–72 life-tables updated to 1976, and Wigle and Mao's 1971 estimates of relative mortality risks by income level. On the basis of this information Wilkins and Adams concluded that the rich live longer than the poor and that the former also enjoy more disability-free years of life. They further observed that "although comprehensive government-administered health-insurance plans have made medical and hospital care available as a right to all Canadians since the late 1960s, this does not mean that socioeconomic-based disparities in health status have been eliminated. Healthfulness of life was directly related to income whether the measure was overall life expectancy, disability-free life or quality-adjusted life expectancy."[87]

While relying heavily upon aggregate proxies to measure the economic status of individuals, the findings of the studies on longevity are congruent with the main body of research evidence on class disparities and health status. Most of these reports have drawn upon prevalence information on findings collected within a brief span of time. Little research attention has been paid in Canada to the impact on health status of social mobility through time or, conversely, to how prolonged or severe ill health may affect an individual's economic circumstances.

Among nine studies drawing upon longitudinal class-related findings, five dealt with the utilization of services, one with public attitudes towards mental illness, two traced changes in health status and one focused on longevity. Two previously noted Saskatchewan reports focusing on structural changes in how health services were provided documented the class-related impact on the selective use of services in Wheatville between 1960 and 1965 and the consequences of medical extra-billing charges between 1966 and 1973.[88] The results of two other longitudinal utilization studies were respectively inconclusive and limited by the research methods used.[89]

Drawing upon survey information and provincial health-insurance records, the Manitoba Longitudinal Study on Aging followed the use of medical and hospital services of 4,558 elderly men and women between 1970 and 1978.[90] While the persons included in this study were relatively homogeneous in terms of income, with 73 per cent living below the official poverty line, low-income compared to high-income elderly persons used fewer medical services annually (5.4 versus 6.1 visits) and were more likely to have been admitted to hospital (23.7 versus 17.2 per cent) during the first two years of the study. More non-users were single, had some degree of mental impairment, and were less well educated. Over a follow-up period of seven years, no association was found between the initial use and non-use of services during the first two years and subsequent rates for hospitalization and mortality.

In relation to public attitudes towards mental illness, C. D'Arcy's 1974 replication of the 1951 survey conducted by E. and J. Cumming in two prairie towns indicated that few changes had occurred and there was little variation in this regard by educational background.[91] In contrast to these relatively stable western communities, Stirling County in Nova Scotia, studied by the Leightons and their colleagues between 1952 and 1970, had become more urbanized, had expanded opportunities for women in service occupations, and experienced a decline in primary industries employing men.[92] During this period the participation of males in the labour force dropped from 76 to 64 per cent, while the rate for women rose from 16 to 27 per cent. The extensive documentation over time of the incidence of depression and anxiety revealed no changes in the rates for these conditions. However, during the interval of almost two decades, a levelling-off by sex occurred, with the rates declining slightly for women and rising for men. The investigators concluded that "in the domains of depression and anxiety ... the increasing number of employed women is relevant to the narrowing gap between men and women in this regard ... employment in the labor force is itself a source of support not only in the economic sense but also in the psychosocial sense."[93]

The Ontario Longitudinal Study on Aging traced the health status of about half of an initial cohort of 2,000 forty-five-year-old men between 1959 and 1978. Most initially reported they were in good health, although the proportion doing so varied directly with income level. Through time, no marked shifts in reported health status occurred for men maintaining a relatively consistent level of income. However, "a change in income was associated with changes in perceived health. That is, a loss of income was strongly associated with a perceived loss of health and a weaker relationship was observed between an increased income and better perceived health." The investigators further concluded that "the data do not support the argument that changes in health for the majority of people lead to income changes."[94]

The most extensive Canadian longitudinal documentation on income-related life changes was reported in 1990 by Wolfson and his co-authors who drew upon a national sample of 545,769 men enrolled in the Canadian Pension Plan.[95] This source lists date of death and draws upon income information from Revenue Canada. While not accounting for family size and regional income differences, if all of the men in this large cohort had had the life expectancy of wage earners in the highest income bracket, the overall survival rate would have risen by 8 per cent. Lower mortality rates were also found to be co-associated for men who had higher incomes earlier in their careers, an improvement in income level over time, later retirement, and had married.

Taken together, the findings for medical care, health status, and longevity reveal that different opportunities, health risks, and life chances exist in Canada for the poor and the non-poor. While these problems have been acknowledged by three federal ministers of Health who held office for sixteen years between 1972 and 1988, none has directly addressed the issue of how persistent class inequities in health care and life chances were to be reduced.[96] Significant improvements in health status, particularly for the poor, are clearly feasible, but whether they will be realized soon in the context of existing class divisions in Canada is another matter.

OPTIONS FOR CHANGE

In their assessments of health care in Western industrialized nations, various commentators have called for radical changes or, less often, have accepted the status quo as inevitable and unalterable. The most popular, yet simplistic, approach is to select a villain, usually the medical profession, and to assume that if its powers were curtailed, greater equity would be achieved. This stance, however, ignores the deeper social and economic roots perpetuating health-care inequalities. Ivan Illich, for instance, in *Medical Nemesis* attacks the medical establishment as "a major threat to health."[97] Its dismantling, he contends, would achieve greater individual autonomy and equity in health care. Illich's homily, however, ignores how broader forces influence health status, and he is singularly silent about how his utopia is to be achieved.

Contrasting with this search for a simpler state of affairs is the neo-Marxist perspective of writers such as V. Navarro and H. Waitzkin, which recognizes that few significant changes will be made in the health system unless they are preceded by a broader realignment of society itself.[98] At least for Canadian society, the necessary preconditions for such a revolution are neither evident nor probable in the period ahead. The traditional proletariat is virtually non-existent in Canada. The advocates of the working class who are heard are relatively powerless and ignored. When they speak on issues such as poverty and illness, the demand is generally for more benefits for their own members rather than for a restructured society that would eliminate the "underclass."

Opposed to the advocates of one or another "new order" who call for a dismantling or a radical restructuring of the health system and/or society are those observers who admonish us to accept the status quo since relevant changes are unlikely and health reforms would yield only marginal gains. In terms of the structure of its health system, each nation, according to O.W. Anderson, gets its "just deserts." Referring to the United States, he accepts as equitable the perpetuation of a two-class system of health care. "If this country will fund a generously proportioned system of options for the well-off and comprehensive services for the badly off, it can have both dynamism and equity."[99]Under such conditions dynamism may indeed be achieved, but Anderson's notion of equity is tautological.

For his part, E. Ginsberg concludes that major health reform, even if it could be realized, would achieve a marginal utility in the benefits actually gained. Rather than extending health services, or pushing for "pie in the sky" reforms, public expectations should be moderated.[100] In advocating that nations should learn to live within their means, he ignores the possibility that this is now being done within a broad range of differently structured societies.

How relevant are these contrasting solutions and assessments of health care to the Canadian scene? Those entailing a dismantling or a radical restructuring are improbable courses of action, while the regressive cynicism inherent in assuming an inequitable status quo in unjust and unacceptable.

In light of the information reviewed on how Canada's class structure influences its health system, no substantial change can be expected unless this emanates from a broader realignment of economic opportunities and class power. The introduction of national health insurance and its operation over the past two decades have not fundamentally altered the pre-existing inequities shaped by this country's class structure. While some features of the health system have changed, such as its growing rationalization, these have been institutional palliatives in terms of redressing class-influenced health disparities.

The dominant forces at work in Canadian society during the remainder of the century will likely entrench even further the already sharp class demarcation evident in the health system. Four matters in particular will contribute to this outcome. These are a slowdown in the rate of growth of health expenditures, a changing demographic profile, evolving constitutional arrangements between the federal and provincial governments, and the free-trade deal negotiated with the United States. The first of these will result from the growing momentum in Canada and other Western nations towards greater cost containment and the imposition of an even tighter financial ceiling on health expenditures.[101] These steps, reflected in legislative revisions in fiscal cost-sharing arrangements between 1977 and 1992, will serve to reduce the margin of flexibility and limit the scope of mounting broad positive measures for especially disadvantaged groups. At the same time, the medical profession's militancy over income could rise again, with concomitant pressures to levy discriminatory extra-billing charges, whose known impact limits the care received by the poor and the socially disadvantaged.

Canada's changing demography, a falling birth-rate, and a growing number of the elderly will have a powerful impact not only on the demand for care but also on the social circumstances under which such care is provided. As a majority of the growing number of elderly Canadians will likely continue to live below the poverty line or on low incomes, they will be disproportionately affected as a group in the receipt of health benefits if the scope of these services is eroded or chipped away by user charges. Three reports, drawing upon official health-insurance records for Alberta, Saskatchewan, and Ontario, have shown that when additional health charges are collected, or even if there is a possibility of this being done, the volume of services is reduced among the elderly on public welfare or on low incomes.[102]

Throughout much of its history Canada has been engaged in a simmering constitutional debate that has on occasion divisively boiled over about whether the nation should become more of a centralized state or a looser federation binding together the more powerful provinces. In the realm of social security and national health insurance, these contrasting views surfaced in the advisory reports of the early 1940s and were central to the post-war proposals that were sharply rejected by the strong central provinces, Quebec and Ontario, as an infringement of matters falling under provincial jurisdiction. The debate then turned on whether there should be a program of state medicine or national health insurance, and whether the federal government should exercise full authority or the plans should be provincially run, assisted by federal grants. Opposing these post-war federal proposals, the provinces sought a transfer of tax points from Ottawa, which then controlled about two-thirds of the country's taxation revenues. The compromise that evolved was the gradual phasing-in of a national health-insurance program, culminating in the 1966 Medical Care Act. This legislation set minimum universal standards acceptable to but also adaptable by the provinces. As Marsh had forecast with considerable prescience in 1943, this course of action provided "no guarantee that some provinces would not lag behind," coupled with "the danger of considerable divergence in scope and type of coverage."[103]

Four decades later this prediction has proved to be valid. With Ottawa now controlling only a third of the country's taxation revenues, national health insurance has become a loosely woven patchwork quilt of provincial plans. According to Monique Begin, who stepped down as minister of Health in 1984, "at the head of this institution there is no big boss; no one founder. At the top is a precarious balance of three key players: the provincial governments, the medical associations and the federal government. Any ... [can] ... decide to block the smooth operation of the system or change the rules or the nature of the game. None is above or below the other."[104]

In more recent times, the clash over jurisdictional authority was also brought to a head by the 1976 election in Quebec of a separatist provincial government and sharp opposition to the patriation of the constitution from Great Britain. During the first half of 1981, when the Constitution Act was before Parliament, it was adamantly rejected by the official opposition party and a majority of the provincial governments on the grounds that its terms infringed on programs coming under provincial jurisdiction and would considerably extend the powers of the federal government.

As the debate over the terms of the 1981 Constitution Act proceeded, it became apparent that if the views of the provinces prevailed, then there would be both greater diversity and an entrenchment of sharp regional disparities in the amount and types of health services available to Canadians, depending upon where they lived in the nation. In contrast, the federal government's position was that the proposed legislation could serve as a powerful catalyst to reduce regional differences in the provision of public services.

In the accord reached on 5 November 1981 a compromise was reached between these polar positions, one whose repercussions continue to be a source of much divisiveness. The broad terms of the Constitution Act and the Charter of Rights were ratified with limiting conditions allowing the provinces to opt out of sections if such decisions were endorsed by provincial legislatures. The effect of this accord confirmed the federal structure of the nation, but created a constitutional structure skewed in favour of preserving regional powers and disparities.

In terms of its reform implications, the accord enunciated for the first time in Canada a legislative concern to promote "equal opportunities for the well-being of Canadians" and "to reduce disparities in opportunities."[105] In the past, major judicial decisions on constitutional matters have reflected a conservative Anglo-Canadian tradition based on legal precedents. The 1981 accord established the basis for the development of a new and evolving body of jurisprudence based directly upon legislative priorities set within the nation. But such changes relating to the legal interpretation of the equality clauses of the new constitution, if they are forthcoming, will only evolve slowly and are subject to provincial powers of veto, as in the case of Quebec's rejection of the portability of health-insurance benefits specified in the 1984 Canada Health Act.

Adapting to this evolving realignment of power in the operation of national health insurance, the federal government in recent years, with the exception of the 1984 Canada Health Act, has sought the high moral ground of developing by consensus initiatives of national concern, such as strategies to control the spread of AIDS and health promotion geared to change individual lifestyles. Conversely, conservative-minded federal officials have been little inclined to disrupt a good public image by dealing directly or substantially with problems deemed to be too contentious or that can be seen as coming under the jurisdiction of the provinces. Falling by the wayside here has been the development of clearly enunciated national policies concerning the supply and distribution of health manpower, the marshalling of documentation about cost-efficient alternatives in providing health services, and ways of addressing the health needs and reducing the inequitable life-chances of the poor and the socially disadvantaged. Except for occasional rhetorical asides, it can be anticipated that the issue of poverty and ill health will continue, in T.H. Marshall's phrase, to remain "invisible" at the national level of social-policy formulation.

The impact on this country's health system of the free-trade agreement negotiated between Canada and the United States during the late 1980s will be unknown for some time. However, the closer economic union may serve in time to weaken east-west links within Canada in favour of north-south ties and lead to a more regressive cutting-edge in this country's taxation policies, and the pressures towards the privatization and containment of social-benefit programs may limit the development of new national measures in the health sector. These trends are buttressed by a prevailing neo-conservative political philosophy in major Western nations that calls for a capping or reduction of state responsibility for social programs such as education, welfare, and health care. Stressing a more active role for the individual and a strengthening of family cohesion, this community-development approach places more responsibility on the individual and local services to fend for themselves in meeting basic social needs.

This philosophy is in part reflected in the regressive impact of increases in taxation introduced between 1984 and 1989. As a result of the combination of changes in income and consumption (sales and excise) taxes, capital-gains exemptions, and the erosion of family benefits, lower-income earners during this period paid on average more than double the proportion of their incomes on taxes than high-income earners.[106] Simultaneously, relative to having a competitive economic environment favourable to international business interests, Canada's ranking among thirty-two nations rose from being eleventh in 1986 to fourth in 1988.[107]

In terms of the prospects of reducing class-related inequities in health care across Canada, there were few encouraging signs at the beginning of the 1990s. Among these, there was a growing recognition that reordering the basic features of Canadian society, such as assuring income adequacy, providing a safer ecosystem, and improving political and cultural well-being, were basic prerequisites for the attainment of better health for all Canadians.[108] Despite these calls for reform, comparable to those advocated by Leonard Marsh in the 1930s, the momentum towards the greater rationalization of health services, evolving demographic shifts, the 1981 constitutional accord coupled with the ensuing protacted unity debate, and closer economic ties with the United States all heralded at best the retention of the status quo or, more likely, movement towards a class structure even more regressive in its consequences for health care.

The Royal Commission on Health Services concluded in 1964 that "we cannot ignore the unequal distribution of resources ...; to meet our health needs ... we are convinced that, however much we prefer voluntary to public action, nothing but public action and support at every level of government can correct the imbalance."[109] This verdict is still valid. It raises the dilemma of which of two contradictory national ethical imperatives is more important in Canadian society. On the one hand, there is a deep-rooted tradition of populism that has fostered strong provincial government and vigorous local initiatives. On the other hand, these values run counter to the attempts of a central authority to achieve reasonable equity through universal-benefit programs.

What is evolving in Canada is an attempt to achieve the best of both worlds. But because the basic premises of the concepts of the universality of benefits and greater public empowerment in setting regional and local priorities are incompatible, these purposes will be neither set aside nor fully achieved in the present structure of Canadian society. Indeed, it is unclear how both can be fully recognized in any nation.

NOTES

1 Canada, Commons, *Debates*, third session, 26th Parliament, 5 April 1965, 2.

2 M. Lalonde, "Health Services Managers or Managers of Health?" *Journal of Health Administration Education* 6 (1988): 76.

3 "Health Care Plan Satisfactory 84% in Ontario tell Gallup," *Toronto Star*, 11 Apr. 1989, A9; R.J. Blendon, "Three Systems: A Comparative Survey," *Health Management Quarterly* 11 (1989): 2–10; and R.J. Blendon and H. Taylor, "Datawatch: Views on Health Care: Public Opinion in Three Nations," *Health Affairs* 8 (1989): 149–57.

4 P. Townsend and N. Davidson, eds., *Inequalities in Health* (Black Report), and M. Whitehead, The Health Divide (London: Penguin Books 1988); Canada, *Achieving Health for All: A Framework for Health Promotion* (Epp Report) (Ottawa: Supply and Service Canada 1986); Ontario Health Review Panel, *Toward a Shared Direction for Health in Ontario* (Evans Report) (Toronto: Government of Ontario 1987); Minister's Advisory Group on Health Promotion, *Health Promotion Matters in Ontario* (Podborski Report) (Toronto: Government of Ontario 1987); and Panel on Health Goals for Ontario, *Health for All Ontario* (Spasoff Report) (Toronto: Government of Ontario 1987).

5 O. Adams and R. Wilkins, *Social Inequalities in Health in Canada: A Review of Current Research, Data and Methodological Issues* (Ottawa: Health

Division, Statistics Canada 1988), 22 pp, mimeo; C. D'Arcy, *Reducing Inequalities in Health*, Health Services and Promotion Branch Working Paper (Ottawa: Health and Welfare Canada 1988); K.R. Grant, "The Inverse Care Law in Canada: Differential Access under Universal Free Health Insurance", in B.S. Bolaria and H.D. Dickinson, eds., *Sociology of Health Care in Canada* (Toronto: Harcourt Brace Jovanovich 1988), 118–34; G. Grenier, "Health Care Costs in Canada: Past and Future Trends," in F. Vaillancourt, Research Coordinator, *Income Distribution and Economic Security in Canada*, vol. 1, Research Studies of the Royal Commission on the Economic Union and Development Prospects for Canada (Toronto: University of Toronto Press 1985), 251–82; P. Manga, "Equality of Access and Inequalities in Health Status: Policy Implications of a Paradox," in D. Coburn, C. D'Arcy, G. Torrance, and P.K.-M. New, eds., *Health and Canadian Society* (Markham: Fitzhenry and Whiteside 1987), 637–48; I. Rootman, "Inequities in Health: Sources and Solutions," *Health Promotion* 26 (1988): 2–8; and R. Wilkins, "Health Inequalities in Canada: Some Policy Implications," *Heart Health Inequalities*, Report of a Workshop on Heart Health Inequalities in Canada, Montreal, 3 December 1987, 5–10.

6 Canadian Council on Social Development, "Towards Social Reform – WIN: Work and Income in the Nineties," *Social Development Overview* 4 (1986): 1–18; Canada, *Report of the Royal Commission on the Economic Union and Development Prospects for Canada* (Ottawa: Supply and Services Canada 1985), 2:545–53; K.G. Banting, "The Welfare State and Inequality in the 1980s," *Canadian Review of Sociology and Anthropology* 24 (1987): 309–38; and A. Freeman, "Household Incomes Fall 1.5%," *Globe and Mail*, 19 March 1992, A1, A6.

7 T. Marshall, *The Right to Welfare and Other Essays* (London: Heinemann Educational Books 1981), 46.

8 Canada, *Financing of Health Services*, paper prepared by the Government of Canada for the Eighth Commonwealth Health Ministers Meeting, Nassau, Bahamas, 13–17 Oct. 1986 (London: Commonwealth Secretariat 1986); and Canada, Commons, *Debates*, second session, 34th Parliament, 4 April 1989, 30.

9 M. Begin, *Medicare: Canada's Right to Health* (Montreal: Optimum Publishing 1987, English translation 1988), 193, 54.

10 Canada, Commons, *Debates*, first session, 27th Parliament, 12 July 1966, 7549.

11 Ibid., 7545, 7544–5, 7546, 7547, 10,769.

12 Canada, *Royal Commission on Health Services* (Hall Report) (Ottawa: Queen's Printer 1964), 1:493.

13 Canada, Commons, *Debates*, second session, 33rd Parliament, 20 May 1988, 15,675; J. Simpson, "Compared with the U.S. Health System,

Canada's Model Wins Handily," *Globe and Mail*, 7 June 1991, A 14.

14 Organisation for Economic Co-operation and Development, *The Future of Social Protection* (Social Policy Studies no. 6, Paris: OECD 1988), 42.

15 Canada, Commons, *Debates*, 6 Dec. 1966, 10,773, 10,773–75.

16 Ibid., 21 June 1966, 6721.

17 Canada, *1984–85 Canada Health Act Annual Report* (Ottawa: Supply and Services Canada 1986), 19–21.

18 R. Plain, "Charging the Sick: Observations on the Economic Aspects of Medical Social Policy Reforms," *Medicare: The Decisive Year*. Conference Proceedings Series no. 3 (Ottawa: Canadian Centre for Policy Alternatives 1984), 26–61.

19 M.G. Taylor, "The Canadian Health Care System 1974–1984," in R.G. Evans and G.J. Stoddart, eds., *Medicare at Maturity: Achievements, Lessons and Challenges* (Calgary: University of Calgary Press 1986), 36.

20 M. Begin, *Medicare* (1987), 182; and *1984–85 Canada Health Act Annual Report* (1986), 19–21.

21 Letter from Dr T–, Mar. 1989; see also B. Joy, "Doctors' Fees for Services," *Oakville Beaver*, 22 Mar. 1989, CL2.

22 *Globe and Mail*, 4 Oct. 1988, A4.

23 D.J. Savoie, *Regional Economic Development: Canada's Search for Solutions* (Toronto: University of Toronto Press 1986), 107–33.

24 Canadian Council on Social Development, "Social Statistics," *Social Development Overview* 6 (Spring 1989): 8.

25 Canada, *Minutes of Proceedings and Evidence of the Standing Committee on Health, Welfare and Social Affairs Respecting Bill C-3 Canada Health Act* (Ottawa: House of Commons 1984); and E.M. Hall, *Canada's National-Provincial Health Program for the 1980s: A Commitment for Renewal* (Saskatoon: Craft Litho Ltd. 1984).

26 T.G. Thall, *Five Perspectives on Health Funding in Canada* (Ottawa: Health and Welfare Canada 1987), 25 pp, mimeo.

27 M.L. Barer and R.G. Evans, "Riding North on a South-bound Horse? Expenditures, Prices, Utilization and Incomes in the Canadian Health Care System," in R.G. Evans and G.J. Stoddart, eds., *Medicare at Maturity: Achievements, Lessons and Challenges* (Calgary: University of Calgary Press 1986), 67.

28 Thall, *Five Perspectives*, 15–16; and Canada, *Medical Care Annual Report 1983* (Ottawa: Supply and Services Canada 1986), 22–3.

29 Canada, *Royal Commission on Health Services*, 237–95 and 521–94.

30 Canadian Council on Social Development, *Social Statistics*, 8; "How Many Doctors Is Too Many?" *Globe and Mail*, 9 December 1991, A5.

31 M.G. Brown, *Caring for Profit: Economic Dimensions of Canada's Health Industry* (Vancouver: Fraser Institute 1987), 107.

32 K.G. Banting, *The Welfare State*, 326–7.

33 Statistics Canada, *Procedures/Technologies by Province, 1984–85*, information provided by Information Production Section, Health Division, June 1989; Canada, *Census/recensement 1986: Census Divisions and Subdivisions* (Ottawa: Statistics Canada 1987), 1–1 to 1–5; and Canada, *Census/Recensement Canada 1986: Total Income Individuals* (Ottawa: Statistics Canada 1989), 3–1 to 3–9.

34 J.R. Jeffery, T.A. Hutchinson, G.S. Arbus, and G.A. Posen, "Kidney Transplantation in Canada, 1981–84," *Canadian Medical Association Journal* 135 (1986): 769–72.

35 Task Force on the Allocation of Health Care Resources, *Health: A Need for Redirection* (Ottawa: Canadian Medical Association 1984), 60.

36 P. McDonough, *The Development and Diffusion of Midtrimester Genetic Amniocentesis*, MSc, University of Toronto 1988, 45–61.

37 M.A.M. de Wachter, "Prenatal Diagnosis," in D.J. Roy and M.A.M. de Wachter, eds., *The Life Technologies and Public Policy* (Montreal: Institute for Research on Public Policy 1986), 87.

38 L.C. Marsh, A.G. Grant, and C.F. Blackler, *Health and Unemployment: Some Studies of Their Relationships*, McGill Social Research Series no. 7 (Montreal 1938), 216, 215.

39 L. Marsh, *Report on Social Security for Canada* (Toronto: University of Toronto Press 1975), xxiii.

40 M. Shore, *The Science of Social Redemption: McGill, the Chicago School, and the Origins of Social Research in Canada* (Toronto: University of Toronto Press 1987).

41 L. Richter, "The Effect of Health Insurance on the Demand for Health Services," *Canadian Journal of Economics and Political Science* 10 (1944): 179–205.

42 Canada, Dominion Bureau of Statistics and Department of National Health and Welfare, *Canadian Sickness Survey, 1950–51*, no. 9, Volume of Health Care for Selected Income Groups (Ottawa: Queen's Printer 1956), 13, 22.

43 Ibid., 17, 22.

44 Those not directly cited include B.J. Darsky, M. Sinai, and S.J. Alexrod, *Comprehensive Medical Services under Voluntary Health Insurance: A Study of Windsor Medical Services* (Cambridge, Mass.: Harvard University Press 1958); K.R. Davidson and E. Davidson, "Healthways in Seaward: A Nova Scotia Fishing Community," *Canadian Journal of Public Health* 67 (1969): 187–91; D.G. Fish, C. Beaudry, and J.J. Day, "Influence of the Social Characteristics of the Family on the Utilization of Health Services," *College of General Practice of Canada Journal* 12 (1966): 34–42; and K.B. Laughton, C.W. Buck, and G.E. Hobbs, "Socio-Economic Status and Illness," *Milbank Memorial Fund Quarterly* 36 (1958): 46–57.

45 D.C. Leighton, J.S. Harding, D.B. Mocklin, A.M. Macmillan, and A.H. Leighton, *The Character of Danger: Psychiatric Symptoms in Selected Communities* (New York: Books 1963), 294.

46 R.F. Badgley and R.W. Hetherington, "Medical Care in Wheatville," *Canadian Journal of Public Health* 52 (1961): 512–17; R.F. Badgley and R.W. Hetherington, "Medical Care and Social Class in Wheatville," *Canadian Journal of Public Health* 53 (1962): 425–31; and R.F. Badgley, R.W. Hetherington, V.L. Matthews, and M. Schulte, "The Impact of Medicare in Wheatville, Saskatchewan: 1960–65," *Canadian Journal of Public Health* 58 (1967): 101–8.

47 Those not directly cited include S. Greenhill, "What Does the Public Want of Health Services?" *Canadian Journal of Public Health* 63 (1972): 108–12; S. Greenhill, "Alberta Health Care Utilization Study: 1968 and 1970," *Canadian Journal of Public Health* 62 (1971): 17–22; G.H. Miller, M. Dear, and D.L. Streiner, "A Model for Predicting Utilization of Psychiatric Facilities," *Canadian Journal of Psychiatry* 34 (1986): 424–30; J. O'Loughlin and J.-F. Boivin, *Indicateurs de santé, facteurs de risque liés au mode de vie et utilisation du système de soins dans la région centre ouest de Montréal*, Quebec Programme de recherche: Recueil de résumés (Québec: Les Publications du Québec 1987), 159–68; Québec, *Et la santé?* tome 2, *Rapport de l'enquête santé Québec 1987* (Québec: Les Publications du Québec 1988), 94; Québec, Rapport de la Commission d'Enquête sur les Services de Santé et les Services Sociaux (Québec: Les Publications du Québec 1988), 73–4, 81–7; and J. Segovia, R.F. Barlett, A.C. Edwards and B. Veitch, *Lifestyle, Health Practices and Utilization of Health Services* (St John's: Memorial University of Newfoundland 1987).

48 P.E. Enterline, J.C. McDonald, A.D. McDonald, L. Davignon, and V. Salter, "Effects of 'Free' Medical Care on Medical Practice – The Quebec Experience," *New England Journal of Medicine* 288 (1973): 1152–5; P.E. Enterline, V. Salter, A.D. McDonald, and J.C. McDonald, "The Distribution of Medical Services before and after 'Free' Medical Care – The Quebec Experience," *New England Journal of Medicine* 289 (1973): 1174–8; A.D. McDonald, J.C. McDonald, N. Steinmetz, P.E. Enterline, and V. Salter, "Physician Services in Montreal before Universal Health Insurance," *Medical Care* 11 (1973): 269–86; A.D. McDonald, J.C. McDonald, V. Salter, and P.E. Enterline, "Effects of Quebec Medicare on Physician Consultation for Selected Symptoms," *New England Journal of Medicine* 291 (1974): 649–52; P.E. Enterline, J.C. McDonald, A.D. McDonald, and V. Henderson, "Physicians' Working Hours and Patients Seen before and after National Health Insurance," *Medical Care* 13 (1975): 95–103; J.R. Hoey and A.D. McDonald, "Hospital Admission before and after Medicare in Quebec," *Medical Care* 16 (1978): 72–

8; E.M. Ricci, P. Enterline, and V. Henderson, "Contacts with Pharmacists before and after 'Free' Medical Care – The Quebec Experience," *Medical Care* 16 (1978): 256–62; and P.E. Enterline, A.D. McDonald, and J.C. McDonald, *Some Effects of Quebec Health Insurance*, DHEW Publication no. (P.H.S.) 79–3238 (Washington 1979).

49 L. Munan, J. Vobecky, and A. Kelly, "Population Health Practices: An Epidemiological Study of the Immediate Effects of a Universal Health Insurance Plan," *International Journal of Health Services* 4 (1974): 285–95.

50 Mathematica Policy Research, Princeton, NJ, *Responses of Canadian Physicians to the Introduction of Universal Medical Care Insurance: The First Five Years in Quebec*, DHEW Publication no. (P.H.S.) 80–3229 (Washington 1980), 9.

51 M.L. Barer and R.G. Evans, *Riding North on a Southbound Horse?* 83–5.

52 N. Steinmetz and J.R. Hoey, "Hospital Emergency Room Utilization in Montreal before and after Medicare: The Quebec Experience," *Medical Care* 16 (1978): 133–9; and Quebec, *Et la santé?* 97.

53 Canada, *Distributional Effects of Health and Educational Benefits* (Ottawa: Statistics Canada 1974; J.A. Boulet and D.W. Henderson, *Distributional and Redistributional Aspects of Government Health Insurance Programs in Canada*, Economic Council of Canada Discussion Paper 146 (Ottawa 1979); T.T.H. Wan and J.H. Broida, "Factors Affecting Variations in Health Services Utilization in Quebec, Canada," *Socioeconomic Planning Sciences* 15 (1981): 231–42; Wan and Broida, "Indicators for Planning of Health Services: Assessing Impacts of Social and Health Care Factors on Population Health," *Socioeconomic Planning Sciences* 17 (1983): 225–34; and Wan and Broida, "Socio-Economic Determinants of Hospital Utilization in Quebec, Canada, 1970–1975," *International Journal of Health Services* 16 (1986): 43–55; G.H. Miller, M. Dear, and D.L. Streiner, *A Model for Predicting Utilization*, 424–30; J. O'Loughlin and J.-F. Boivin, *Indicateurs de santé*, 159–68.

54 Canada, *Distributional Effects of Health*, 49.

55 Those not directly cited include M.L. Barer, P. Manga, E.R. Shillington, and G.C. Siegel, *Income Class and Hospital Use in Ontario* (Toronto: Ontario Economic Council 1982); Department of National Health and Welfare, *Nutrition Canada National Survey* (Ottawa: Information Canada 1973); P. Manga, *The Income Distribution Effect of Medical Insurance in Ontario* (Toronto: Ontario Economic Council 1978); J. Siemiatycki, L. Richardson, and I.B. Pless, "Equality in Medical Care under National Health Insurance in Montreal," *New England Journal of Medicine* 303 (1980): 10–15; N.P. Roos and E. Shapiro, "The Manitoba Longitudinal Study on Aging," *Medical Care* 19 (1981) 644–57; and L.A. Strain, *Physician Utilization and Illness Behaviour in Old Age; Prediction and Process* PhD, University of Toronto 1988.

56 R. Kohn and K.L. White, eds., *Health Care: An International Study* (London: Oxford University Press 1976).

57 R.D. Smith, *Social Class and Health Behaviour*, PhD, University of Toronto 1980.

58 J. Feather, *A Response-Record Discrepancy Study*, WHO International Collaborative Study on Medical Care Utilization, Saskatchewan Study Area Reports, ser. 2, Methodological Studies, Monograph no. 2 (Saskatoon 1972).

59 Siemiatycki, Richardson and Pless, *Equality in Medical Care*, 12.

60 Canada, *Canada Fitness Survey* (Ottawa: Fitness and Amateur Sport 1983); Canada, *Report of the Canadian Health and Disability Survey: 1983–1984* (Ottawa: Supply and Services Canada 1986); Canada, *Canada's Health Promotion Survey: Technical Report* (Ottawa: Supply and Services Canada 1988).

61 Canada, *The Health of Canadians: Report of the Canada Health Survey* (Ottawa: Supply and Services Canada 1987), 174; Canada, *Health and Social Support Survey 1985* (Ottawa: Supply and Services Canada 1987), 75–8, 83.

62 R.W. Broyles, P. Manga, D.A. Binder, D.E. Angus, and A. Charette, "The Use of Physician Services under a National Health Insurance Scheme," *Medical Care*, 21 (1983): 1047; P. Manga, R.W. Broyles, and D. Angus, *The Use of Hospital and Physician Services under a National Health Insurance Program: An Examination of the Canada Health Survey*, University of Ottawa Faculty of Administration Working Paper 83–65 (Ottawa 1983); and P. Manga, "Equality of Access and Inequalities in Health Status: Policy Implications of a Paradox," in D. Coburn, C. D'Arcy, G. Torrance, and P.K.-M. New, eds., *Health and Canadian Society: Sociological Perspectives* (Markham, Ont.: Fitzhenry and Whiteside 1987), 637–48.

63 J.A. Boan, ed., *Proceedings of the Second Canadian Conference on Health Economics: Health Insurance: A Silver Anniversary Appraisal* (Regina: University of Regina 1983), 73.

64 Canadian Council on Social Development, "Toward Social Reform – WIN: Work and Income in the Nineties," *Social Development Overview* 4 (1986): 1–18; and Canada, *Report of the Royal Commission on the Economic Union and Development Prospects for Canada* (Ottawa: Supply and Services Canada 1985), 2:545–53.

65 Those not directly cited include T. Atkinson, B. Blishen, and M. Murray, *Physical Status and Perceived Health Quality* (Toronto: Institute for Behavioural Research 1980); D.I. Hay, *Socioeconomic Status and Health Status: A Study of Males in the Canada Health Survey*, MSc, University of Toronto 1985; Mathematica Policy Research Princeton, *Responses of Canadian Physicians 1980*; N.P. Roos and L.L. Roos, "Surgical Rate Variations: Do They Reflect the Heatlh or Socioeconomic Characteristics of

the Population?" *Medical Care* 20 (1982); 945–58; R.D. Smith, *Social Class and Health Behaviour*; E.L. Snider, "Factors Influencing Health Service Knowledge among the Elderly," *Journal of Health and Social Behavior* 21 (1980): 371–7; N. Steinmetz, *Hospital Emergency Room Utilization*; and W.M. Warner, "Lower Socioeconomic Groups and Preventive Public Health Programs: A Problem of Communication Effectiveness," *Canadian Journal of Public Health* 64 (1973): 562–73.

66 R.G. Beck and J.M. Horne, "Before and after Copayment in Saskatchewan: 1968–71," in R.F. Badgley and R.D. Smith, *User Charges for Health Services* (Toronto: Ontario Council of Health 1979), 121–62.

67 P. Manga, *The Income Distribution Effect of Medical Insurance in Ontario*, Ontario Economic Council Occasional Paper 6 (Toronto 1978).

68 Badgley and Smith, *User Charges*, 166–94.

69 R.F. Badgley, D. Fortin Caron, and M.G. Powell, *Report of the Committee on the Operation of the Abortion Law* (Ottawa: Supply and Services Canada 1977), 388–405.

70 M. LeClair, "The Canadian Health Care System," in S. Andreopoulous, ed., *National Health Insurance: Can We Learn from Canada?* (New York: John Wiley and Sons 1975), 42.

71 Broyles, *The Use of Physician Services*, 1051; and Siemiatycki, *Equality in Medical Care*, 10.

72 L.G. Williams, "Patterns of Family Spending for Personal Health Services in Canada," *Canada's Health and Welfare* 23 (1968): 5–8.

73 J. Ableson, P. Padden, and C. Strohmenger, *Perspectives on Health* (Ottawa: Supply and Services Canada 1983), 13, 109, 110; and Statistics Canada, *Family Expenditure in Canada* (Ottawa: Supply and Services Canada, reports issued between 1972 and 1984).

74 Canada, *Report of the Royal Commission on the Economic Union*, Volume II, 537–615.

75 Canada, Commons, *Debates*, 7545.

76 Canada, *Work Injuries 1983–1985* (Ottawa: Supply and Services Canada 1987); Canada, *Work Injuries 1985–1987* (Ottawa: Supply and Services Canada 1988).

   M.H. Boyle, D.R. Offord, H.G. Hofmann, G.P. Catlin, J.A. Byles, D.T. Cadman, J.W. Crawford, P.S. Links, N.I. Rae-Grant, and P. Szatmari, "Ontario Child Health Study: I. Methodology," *Archives of General Psychiatry* 44 (1987): 826–31; D.R. Offord, J.M. Last, and P.A. Barretta, "A Comparison of the School Performance, Emotional Adjustment and Skill Development of Poor and Middle-Class Children," *Canadian Journal of Public Health* 76 (1985): 174–8; D.R. Offord, M.H. Boyle, P. Szatmari, N.I. Rae-Grant, P.S. Links, D.T. Cadman, J.A. Byles, J.W. Crawford, H.M. Blum, C. Byrne, H. Thomas, and C.A. Woodward, "Ontario Child Health Study: II. Six-Month Prevalence of Disorder and Rates of Service Utilization," *Archives of General Psychia-*

try 44 (1987): 832–6; D.R. Offord, M.H. Boyle, and B.R. Jones, "Psychiatric Disorder and Poor School Performance among Welfare Children in Ontario," *Canadian Journal of Psychiatry* 32 (1987): 518–25; and C.P. Shah, M. Kahan, and J. Krauser, "The Health of Children of Low-Income Families," *Canadian Medical Association Journal* 137 (1987): 485–90.

C. D'Arcy and C.M. Siddique, "Unemployment and Health: An Analysis of Canada Health Survey Data," *International Journal of Health Services* 15 (1985): 609–35; see also C. D'Arcy, "Unemployment and Health: Data and Implications," *Canadian Journal of Public Health* 77, supp. 1 (1986): 124–31; and L. Soderstrom, "The Effects of Unemployment on the Health of Unemployed Married Women," in J.M. Horne, ed., *Proceedings of the Third Canadian Conference on Health Economics* (Winnipeg: University of Manitoba 1986), 219–58.

Daily Bread Food Bank, *The Kids Are Hungry* (Toronto 1989), 4 pp; M. Desoulniers and M. Beaudry-Darisme, "Les habitudes alimentaires des adultes de trois milieux socio-économiques de la ville de Québec," *Journal of the Canadian Dietetic Association* 39 (1978): 39–45; A.G. Higgins, "Nutritional Status and the Outcome of Pregnancy," *Journal of the Canadian Dietetic Association* 37 (1976): 17–35; O.B. Martinez, "Growth and Dietary Quality of Young French Canadian School Children," *Journal of the Canadian Dietetic Association* 43 (1982): 28–35; A.W. Myres and D. Kroetsch, "The Influence of Family Income on Food Consumption Patterns and Nutrient Intake in Canada," *Canadian Journal of Public Health* 69 (1978): 208–21; and A.D. Sullivan and N.E. Schwartz, "Attitudes, Knowledge and Practice Related to Diet and Cardiovascular Disease," *Journal of the Canadian Dietetic Association* 42 (1981): 169–77.

D.I. Hay, "Socioeconomic Status and Health Status: A Study of Males in the Canada Health Survey," *Social Science and Medicine* 27 (1988): 1317–25; and W.J. Millar and D.T. Wigle, "Socioeconomic Disparities in Risk Factors for Cardiovascular Disease," *Canadian Medical Association Journal* 134 (1986): 127–32.

77 Canada, *The Health of Canadians*, 114, 117, 131.
78 Canada, *Canadian Health and Disability Survey, 1983–1984.*
79 Canada, *Health and Social Support, 1985*, 124–5.
80 Organisation for Economic Co-operation and Development, *Measuring Health Care, 1960–1983: Expenditures, Costs and Performance* (Paris 1985); and World Bank, *World Development Report 1983* (New York: Oxford University Press 1983).
81 M. Lalonde, *Health Services Managers*, 78; Canada, *Achieving Health for All: A Framework for Health Promotion* (Ottawa: Supply and Services 1986), 4.

82 Those not directly cited include O.B. Adams, *Health and Economic Activity* (Ottawa: Supply and Services Canada 1981); W.J. Millar, "Sex Differentials in Mortality by Income Level in Urban Canada," *Canadian Journal of Public Health* 74 (1983): 329–34; E.S. Nichols and M.H. Smith, "Suicide and Socioeconomic Indicators," *Chronic Diseases in Canada* 3 (1982): 63–4; A.-M. Ugnat and E. Mark, "Life Expectancy by Age, Sex and Income Level," *Chronic Diseases in Canada* 6 (1985): 12–13; and D.T. Wigle, "The Distribution of Cancer in Two Canadian Cities," *Canadian Journal of Public Health* 68 (1977): 463–8.

83 A. Billette and G.B. Hill, *Inégalités sociales de mortalité au Canada* (Ottawa: Health and Welfare Canada 1977).

84 R.P. Gallagher, W.J. Threlfall, P.P. Band, J.J. Spinelli, and A.J. Coldman, *Occupational Mortality in British Columbia: 1950–1978 (Ottawa: Supply and Services Canada 1986).

85 D.T. Wigle and Y. Mao, *Mortality by Income Level in Urban Canada* (Ottawa: Health Protection Branch, Health and Welfare Canada 1980), 1.

86 R. Wilkins, "Health Expectancy by Local Area in Montreal: A Summary of Findings," *Canadian Journal of Public Health* 77 (1986): 216–20; O'Loughlin and Brown, *Indicators de santé*, 159–68; City of Toronto, *Healthy Toronto 2000: A Discussion Paper* (Toronto: Board of Health 1987), 47–9.

87 R. Wilkins and O.B. Adams, "Health Expectancy in Canada, Late 1970s: Demographic, Regional and Social Dimensions," in D. Coburn, C. D'Arcy, G. Torrance and P. K.-M. New, eds., *Health and Canadian Society: Sociological Perspectives* (Markham, Ont.: Fitzhenry and Whiteside 1987), 52; see also R. Wilkins, *Health Status in Canada 1926–1976*, Institute for Research on Public Policy Occasional Paper no. 13 (Montreal 1980); and R. Wilkins and C.B. Adams, *Healthfulness of Life*, The Institute for Research on Public Policy (Montreal 1983).

88 Badgley, Hetherington, Matthews, and Schulte, *Impact of Medicare in Wheatville*, 101–8; Beck and Horne, *Before and After Copayment*, 121–62.

89 J. Trainor, K. Boydell, and R. Tibshirani, "Short-Term Economic Change and the Utilization of Mental Health Facilities in a Metropolitan Area," *Canadian Journal of Psychiatry* 32 (1986): 379–83; Enterline, *Effects of "Free" Medical Care*.

90 N.P. Ross and E. Shapiro, "The Manitoba Longitudinal Study on Aging: Preliminary Findings on Health Care Utilization by the Elderly," *Medical Care* 19 (1981): 644–57; and E. Shapiro and N.P. Roos, "Elderly Nonusers of Health Care Services: Their Characteristics and Their Health Outcomes," *Medical Care* 23 (1985): 247–57.

91 E. Cumming and J. Cumming, *Closed Ranks: An Experiment in Mental Health Education* (Cambridge: Harvard University Press 1957); and C. D'Arcy, "Opened Ranks? Blackfoot Revisited," in D. Coburn, C.

D'Arcy, G. Torrance, and P.K.-M. New, eds., *Health and Canadian Society: Sociological Perspectives* (Markham: Fitzhenry and Whiteside 1987), 280–94.

92 Leighton, *The Character of Danger*; and J.M. Murphy, A.M. Sobel, R.K. Neff, D.C. Oliver, and A.H. Leighton, "Stability of Prevalence: Depression and Anxiety Disorders," *Archives of General Psychiatry* 41 (1984): 990–7.

93 J.M. Murphy, "Trends in Depression and Anxiety: Men and Women," *Acta Psychiatrica Scandinavica* 73 (1986): 124.

94 J.P. Hirdes, K.S. Brown, and W.F. Forbes, "The Association between Self-Reported Income and Perceived Health Based on the Ontario Longitudinal Study of Aging," *Canadian Journal on Aging* 5 (1986): 201; Hirdes, Brown and Forbes, *Income and Perceived Health*, 202.

95 M. Wolfson, G. Rowe, J.F. Gentleman and M. Tomiak, *Earnings and Death – Effects over a Quarter Century* (Toronto: Canadian Institute for Advanced Research 1990).

96 Lalonde, *Health Services Managers*, 78; Canada, *Achieving Health for All*, 4; and M. Begin, "Health: An Integral Part of Human Development," *Canadian Journal of Public Health* 69 (1978): 273–4.

97 I. Illich, *Medical Nemesis: The Expropriation of Health* (Toronto: McClelland and Stewart 1975).

98 V. Navarro, *Medicine under Capitalism* (New York: Prodist 1976); V. Navarro, *Class Struggle, the State and Medicine* (New York: Prodist 1978); and H. Waitzkin, *The Second Sickness: Contradictions of Capitalist Health Care* (New York: Free Press 1983).

99 O.W. Anderson, *Health Care: Can There be Equity? The United States, Sweden and England* (New York: John Wiley and Sons 1972), 210.

100 E. Ginzberg, *The Limits of Health Reform: The Search for Realism* (New York: Basic Books 1977).

101 Organisation for Economic Co-operation and Development, *The Future of Social Protection*, Social Policy Studies no. 6 (Paris 1988), 41–6.

102 Plain, *Charging the Sick*, 26–61; Beck and Horne, *Before and after Copayment*, 122–62; and R.F. Badgley and R.D. Smith, *User Charges for Health Services*, 166–94.

103 Marsh, *Report on Social Security for Canada*, 189.

104 Begin, *Medicare: Canada's Right to Health*, 188.

105 Canada, *Constitution Act 1982*.

106 D.P. Ross and R. Shillington, "Lower- and Middle-Income Earners Still Bear Brunt of Taxes," *Social Development Overview* 6 (1989): 1–4.

107 J. Simpson, "Competitive Edges," *Globe and Mail*, 21 July 1989, A6.

108 City of Toronto, *Advocacy for Basic Health Prerequisites: Departmental Policy Paper* (Toronto: Department of Public Health 1991) and On-

tario, *Working Document-Goals and Strategic Priorities: Ministry of Health* (Toronto: Ministry of Health 1992).
109 Canada, *Royal Commission on Health Services*, 1:9.

Contributors

ROBIN F. BADGLEY is a professor in the Department of Behavioural Science, Faculty of Medicine, at the University of Toronto. He has chaired two national inquiries for the government of Canada, on the operation of the abortion law (1975–77) and on sexual offences against children (1980–84). Between 1977 and 1984 he was a member of the Pan American Health Organization's Advisory Committee on Medical Research, and he also served (1985–87) as a consultant on foreign aid for health to the Commonwealth Secretariat (London). With co-author Samuel Wolfe he has written two books: *Doctors' Strike: Medical Care and Conflict in Saskatchewan* (1967) and *The Family Doctor* (1973).

JAY CASSEL was born in New York City and later lived in Montreal and Ottawa. He received his BA in history from Oxford University, an MA from Queen's University, Kingston, and a PhD from the University of Toronto. He has worked as a post-doctoral fellow at York University, Toronto, and has written on a variety of topics in medical history and Canadian social history. His publications include *The Secret Plague: Venereal Disease in Canada, 1838–1939*, which won the Hannah Medal of the Royal Society of Canada. At present he is an assistant professor of history at York University.

TERRY COPP is professor of history and chair of the department at Wilfrid Laurier University in Waterloo, Ontario. He is the author of a number of books and articles on Canadian social history as well as Canadian military history, including *Battle Exhaustion: Soldiers and Psychiatrists in the Canadian Army, 1939–1945* (co-authored with Bill McAndrew), from which this essay is drawn.

RAISA DEBER is professor of health administration in the Faculty of Medicine, Division of Community Health, University of Toronto. She has lectured and written widely on Canadian politics and health policy, medical decision-making, and technology assessment. Her current research projects include an analysis of the development and implementation of the Canada Health Act and a study using interactive videodisc to facilitate shared decision-making between patient and provider. Her recent books include *Managed Care in Canada* (1991), *Restructuring Canada's Health Services System: How Do We Get There from Here?* (1992), and *Case Studies in Canadian Health Policy and Management* (in press).

COLIN D. HOWELL is a professor of history at Saint Mary's University in Halifax, where he is also engaged in the Atlantic Canada Studies Program and a founding member of the Gorsebrook Research Institute. Dr Howell has published widely in the history of the Maritime region and is the author of *A Century of Care: A History of the Victoria General Hospital in Halifax 1887–1987*. At present Dr Howell is co-editor of the *Canadian Historical Review* and a member of the advisory board of the *Canadian Bulletin of Medical History*.

STEPHEN J. KUNITZ is a professor in the Department of Community and Preventive Medicine at the University of Rochester School of Medicine and Dentistry, Rochester, New York. He received a BA in English literature, an MA in the history of science and medicine, and a PhD in sociology, all from Yale University, and an MD from the University of Rochester. He has done research in the history and sociology of medicine.

DESMOND MORTON is a professor of history at the University of Toronto and principal of Erindale College in Mississauga. A graduate of the Collège Militaire Royal de St-Jean, the Royal Military College, Oxford, and the University of London, he is the author of twenty-three books, including *A Short History of Canada*, *The Military History of Canada* (with Glenn Wright), *Winning the Second Battle: Canadian Veterans and the Return to Civilian Life, 1915–1930*, and (with J.L. Granatstein) *Marching to Armageddon: Canadians and the Great War, 1914–1919*.

C. DAVID NAYLOR is a general internist and director of the clinical epidemiology program at Sunnybrook Health Science Centre, a University of Toronto teaching hospital. His primary academic interests are centred on clinical and health-services research in the cardiovascular field. However, he has also published in health policy and social history of medical care, including a monograph, *Private Practice, Public Payment: Canadian Medicine and the Politics of Health Insurance, 1911–1966* (1986).

EUGENE VAYDA is Professor Emeritus of Health Administration and Medicine in the Faculty of Medicine, University of Toronto, where he has served as associate dean of Community Health. He has lectured and written widely on the Canadian health-care system and has carried out research on organization, financing, and payment for health-care services; physician attitudes and behaviour; medical-practice guidelines; and emergency services. Dr Vayda is currently doing comparative studies of health-care systems in the United States and Canada.

SAMUEL WOLFE is currently Professor Emeritus of Public Health at the Columbia University School of Public Health in New York City. He worked as a country doctor in Saskatchewan for seven years and then pursued further training at the University of Saskatchewan and Columbia University before returning to Canada, where he was a commissioner of the Saskatchewan Medical Care Plan (1962–66) and medical director of the Saskatoon Community Clinic (1962–68). Dr Wolfe remained active in the development of community-health programs in the USA and returned to Columbia in mid–1975 to chair the Division of Health Administration in the School of Public Health. He retired in 1991. He and Robin F. Badgley have collaborated and published together for close to thirty years, authoring two books and many articles.

JUDITH YOUNG received her early nursing training at the Hospital for Sick Children, Great Ormond Street, London, England. She has worked at HSC Toronto as a head nurse. Since 1980 Ms Young has been a tutor in the Faculty of Nursing, University of Toronto.